IMMUNOLOGY

made ridiculously simple

Massoud Mahmoudi, DO, PhD, FACOI, FAOCAI, FACP, FCCP, FAAAAI

President
American Osteopathic College of
Allergy and Immunology

Clinical Professor
Department of Medicine
University of California San Franciso

Adjunct Professor
Department of Medicine
School of Osteopathic Medicine
Rowan University
Stratford, New Jersey

Adjunct Professor
Department of Medicine
San Francisco College of Osteopathic Medicine
Touro University
Vallejo, California

Editor/Author of:
Allergy and Asthma, The Basics to Best Practices, Springer, 2019
Allergy and Asthma: Practical Diagnosis and Management (Ed-2), Springer, 2016
Challenging Cases in Rheumatology and Diseases of the Immune System, Springer, 2012
Challenging Cases in Pulmonology, Springer, 2011
Challenging Cases in Allergic and Immunologic Disease of the Skin, Springer, 2010
Challenging Cases in Allergy and Immunology, Springer, 2009

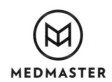

MEDMASTER

ISBN13 #978-0-940780-89-7

Made in the United States of America

Published by
MedMaster, Inc.
P.O. Box 640028
Miami, FL 33164
Cover image by Richard March

To the memory of my father, Mohammad H. Mahmoudi, and to my mother, Zohreh, my wife, Lily, and my son, Sam, for their sincere support and encouragement

Preface

Immunology is the fascinating science of the immune system. Learning this complex subject, however, has never been easy; most immunology textbooks cover too much detail, such as animal studies, that although important are not clinically relevant. Also, while newer textbooks have many diagrams, they usually lack simple visual aids for many of the complex points; at times the reader needs to explore several textbooks to understand the same topic.

An understanding of immunology needs comprehensive study, but we first must comprehend the clinically relevant material in a simple and direct format. I wrote this book to explain simply the common topics in immunology that a student of medicine needs to know.

With simplicity in mind, I found the MedMaster Made Ridiculously Simple series the right medium for teaching a complex subject in a simple style. I was already familiar with the MedMaster series while in my medical training, having owned at least 5 books of the series before approaching Dr. Stephen Goldberg, the publisher. As in other books in this series, I employ visual aids, including cartoons, and a style of writing that includes easy-to-understand, clinically relevant information and fewer details of irrelevant subjects.

This book consists of 10 chapters. The first 3 are basic immunology, and the remaining 7 are relevant clinical chapters. I have tried to include only the need-to-know information but have gone into somewhat more detail in some sections for better understanding and clarification of the subject.

I am indebted to Dr. Goldberg for dedicating his time to make the Made Ridiculously Simple series available for the last 30 years. He closely monitors the writing and its content to maintain the high quality of this fascinating collection. I also express my gratitude to Phyllis Goldenberg for her wonderful proofreading of this manuscript.

I not only urge and recommend this book to all my previous and present students, residents, and fellows, but to all students of medicine. Use this book as a study aide and supplement to your reference immunology textbook. I hope that I have accomplished the goal of this series and have made this book a useful addition. Please feel free to contact me at allergycure@sbcglobal.net. I will use your feedback to improve future editions.

Massoud Mahmoudi

Contents

CONTENTS

PART I. BASIC IMMUNOLOGY

CHAPTER 1. THE WORLD OF THE IMMUNE SYSTEM

Our **immune system** protects us from the invasion of foreign organisms and substances. Invaders include living organisms; microbial toxins and other microbial byproducts; and other foreign substances, such as pollens, pet danders, and chemicals like those used in manufacturing drugs and cosmetics. Our protective status, **immunity**, consists of two distinct types: **innate (natural)** and **adaptive (acquired)**. Although each type of immunity has its own duties in the fight against the invaders, both types work in concert to eliminate the offending agent and return the body to its healthy balance.

INNATE IMMUNITY

Think of innate immunity (natural immunity) as the first line of defense against microbial and non-microbial substances. This type of immunity does not require memory. In other words, the components of this system can react on first exposure to the invading organism or non-microbial substance. The players of this system work in various ways:

- **Physical barrier.** The skin and the mucosal linings of the respiratory and gastrointestinal tract are physical barriers that prevent entrance of organisms into the body. Trauma, such as mechanical injury or burns, breaks these protective barriers and makes them vulnerable to colonization and growth of bacteria. Ciliary motion of the respiratory tract mucosa helps remove foreign objects from the respiratory tract.
- **Secretions.** Bodily secretions help trap, wash off, and destroy organisms and other foreign elements. For example, tears and saliva contain **lysozyme**, an enzyme that kills bacteria by breaking the peptidoglycan layer of cell walls. The acidic character of sweat (due to lactic acid) and stomach gastric acid prevent bacterial colonization and growth by destroying acid-labile organisms.
- **Phagocytosis.** Phagocytosis is the mechanism by which host cells engulf and destroy the organism. The sequence of events includes attraction of microorganisms to the cells, followed by binding to

the cell surface receptors, activation of the cell membrane, surrounding the organism by host pseudopods, and, finally, engulfing the organism. The complex of the engulfed organism and the surrounding membrane is known as a **phagosome** (**Fig. 1-1**). Lysosomal vesicles containing various lytic enzymes fuse with the phagosome to form a **phagolysosome**. The lytic enzymes kill and degrade the organism. When the target is too big to engulf, the phagocyte releases its enzyme extracellularly.

There are two main types of phagocytic cell: neutrophils and macrophages.

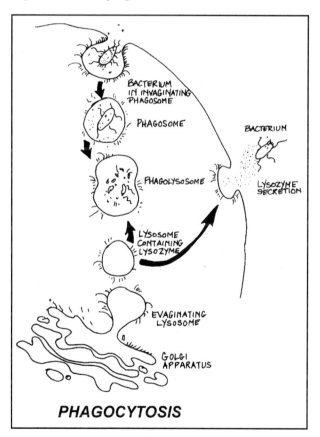

Figure 1-1 (From Goldberg, S., *Clinical Physiology Made Ridiculously Simple*, MedMaster)

- **Neutrophils.** As the predominant white cells in the blood, these multilobed nucleated cells arise from bone marrow (**Fig. 1-2**). After maturation, they are released into the bloodstream, where they live for only 1-2 days. Neutrophilic granules contain lysozyme, which can lyse bacterial cell walls after phagocytosis.

- **Macrophages.** These phagocytic cells derive from monocytes that first form in bone marrow and then enter the bloodstream (**Fig. 1-2**).

Monocytes move to various tissues, where they are called **macrophages** or **histiocytes**. The macrophages of various tissues are named differently, although their functions are basically similar. Some examples are summarized in **Fig. 1-3**.

Natural Killer (NK) Cells

Viruses do not have their own reproductive machinery. They need to infect host cells to propagate. Some intracellular bacteria may also infect host cells. Identification and destruction of these infected cells and some tumor cells are done by a large group of granular lymphocytes known as **Natural Killer (NK) cells**. These cells originate from bone marrow precursors and form 10-15% of peripheral blood lymphocytes.

How does an NK cell identify and destroy the infected cell? It is crucial for the NK cells to destroy infected cells, but not normal cells. They do this through their activating and inhibitory receptors. To prevent the normal host cells from harm, the inhibitory receptors of NK cells bind to a molecule known as **Major Histocompatibility**

FIGURE 1-3

Macrophage Origins

Macrophages	Source
Osteoclast	Bone
Mesangial cells	Kidney
Langerhans cells	Skin
Alveolar macrophages	Lungs
Microglia	Central nervous system
Kupffer cells	Liver
Monocyte	Blood

Complex 1 (MHC-1) on the surface of normal cells. By such binding, the NK cells are inhibited from activation, and the normal host cells are spared from destruction (**Fig. 1-4**). When host cells are infected, the MHC-1 expression is inhibited and, therefore, there is no ligand (a molecule that binds to another) for inhibitory receptors to bind. Then, the NK activating receptor ligands are expressed and bind and destroy the infected cells (**Fig. 1-4**).

NK cell cytoplasmic granules contain **perforin**, an enzyme that makes pores on target cells, and **granzyme**, an enzyme that enters the target cells and causes the cells to

---

Figure 1-2

Figure 1-2 (From Goldberg, S., *Clinical Physiology Made Ridiculously Simple*, MedMaster)

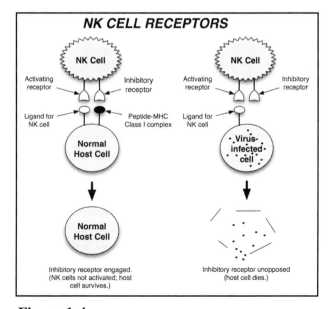

Figure 1-4

commit suicide, a process known as **apoptosis**, or **programmed death**. In addition to lysis of the infected cells, activated NK cells produce **interferon (IFN)-γ**, a **cytokine** that activates macrophages to destroy phagocytized microbes. **Cytokines** (cyto = cell; kinesis = movement) are a group of proteins secreted by different cells in the body to help cell-to-cell communication, as well as inflammatory and immune response reactions. Chemical components of the innate immune system and their functions are summarized in **Fig. 1-5**.

Complement Pathways

Complement is a group of 30 or more plasma and cell surface proteins, mainly synthesized in the liver and distributed in the blood and tissues. They work in concert to fight the invading microorganisms through phagocytosis, inflammation, and lysis (**Fig. 1-6**; complement can is spilling "OIL").

The sequence of events in the complement pathways is as follows: (**Fig. 1-7**):

1. **Activation.** The activation of complement occurs via three distinct pathways: **classical**, **alternative**, and **lectin**.
   - The components of the **classical pathway** include **C1 (C1q, C1r, C1s), C2, C3**, and **C4**. The activation of this pathway is initiated by binding of C1, the first component of the complement system, to the **antigen-antibody** complex. **Antigens** are substances (usually external) that enter

---

FIGURE 1-5

Chemical Components of the Immune System

Proteins	Function
Complement	A group of plasma and cell surface proteins that fights invading organisms through inflammation, phagocytosis, and lysis.
Mannose Binding Protein (MBP)	• Binds to mannose on the surface of bacteria, viruses, and parasites, tagging the organism for phagocytosis. • Activates complement.
C-reactive Protein	Binds to the bacterial surface, acts like **opsonin** (a substance, such as antibody, that binds to an antigen to promote phagocytosis) and activates complement.
Serum amyloid P component	Binds to the surface of bacteria and acts like opsonin.
Lipopolysaccharide Binding Protein (LPS)	Binds to LPS on gram-negative bacteria and makes it the target of a variety of cells, including macrophages.
Cytokines	Secretory proteins produced by lymphocytes and monocytes in response to microbial antigens. Cytokines help: • Cell-to-cell communication • Inflammatory reactions • Immune response reactions
IL (Interleukin) 10	Inhibits macrophage activity.
IL 12, 18, 23	Stimulate NK cells to produce IFN-γ.
IL 15	Promotes inhibition of NK, B, and T cells.
IFN-α and β	• Have antiviral effect. • Stimulate NK cells and promote class I MHC expression.
IFN-γ	Produced by NK cells and activates macrophages.
TGF-β	Stimulates macrophages.

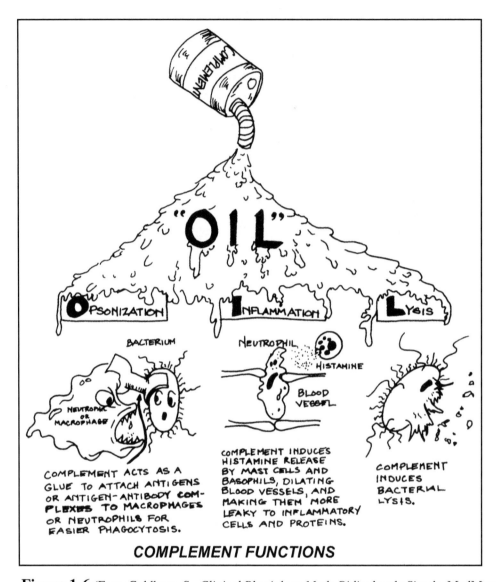

Figure 1-6 (From Goldberg, S., *Clinical Physiology Made Ridiculously Simple*, MedMaster)

the body, bind to an antibody or T cell receptor, and elicit an immune response (discussed in Chapter 2). **Antibody** (also known as immunoglobulin) is a glycoprotein produced by plasma cells in response to antigen (discussed later).

- The components of the **alternative pathway** include **properdin**, **Factor B**, **Factor D**, and **C3**. The activation of this pathway is initiated directly on microbial cell surfaces and is independent of antibodies.

- The activation of the **lectin pathway** starts when a protein known as **mannose binding lectin**

(**MBL**) recognizes mannose residues on the microbial surface. After activation of the **mannose-binding-lectin-associated proteases**, **MASP-1** and **MASP-2**, the remaining part of the pathway is similar to the classical pathway.

2. **Formation of the enzyme C3 convertase.** After several steps of binding and enzymatic events, the enzyme C3 convertase is formed (C3bBb and C4b2a). This enzyme cleaves C3, the most abundant component of the complement system and the center of all complement action, into two components: C3a and C3b (**Fig. 1-7**).

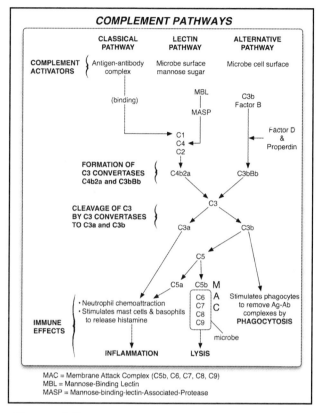

COMPLEMENT PATHWAYS

MAC = Membrane Attack Complex (C5b, C6, C7, C8, C9)
MBL = Mannose-Binding Lectin
MASP = Mannose-binding-lectin-Associated-Protease

Figure 1-7

3. **Opsonization and phagocytosis.** Opsonization is the binding or coating of a microbe by an antibody or a complement. Such binding tags the microbe as a target and identifies it as an easy mark for phagocytosis. The molecule that binds to the microbe, in this case complement, is an opsonin. C3b is an example. Phagocytes that have receptors on their cell surfaces bind to the opsonized molecules and engulf them.

4. **Inflammation.** C3a and C5a are able to attract neutrophils (**chemoattraction**). They also have **anaphylatoxic** activity, in which they bind to and stimulate mast cells and basophils to release the contents of cytoplasmic granules (**degranulation**), including histamine and other vasoactive substances. Binding of histamine to the endothelial layer of capillaries causes their dilation, which allows leakage of fluid and proteins from the blood to the adjacent tissues, leading to inflammation.

5. **Lysis.** C3b cleaves C5 to form C5a and C5b. On the surface of the microbe, C5b forms a complex with C6, C7, C8, and C9 known as **membrane attack complex (MAC)** and causes the lysis of the microbe. **Fig. 1-7** summarizes the events.

ADAPTIVE IMMUNITY

At times, smart bacteria pass undetected through the first line of defense, the innate immunity. Therefore, we need another system of defense, **adaptive (acquired)** immunity. Such immunity can distinguish one specific microbe from another. In addition, adaptive immunity develops memory for subsequent exposure to the same organism.

There are two types of adaptive immunity: **humoral immunity** and **cell-mediated immunity**. The main cells that mediate adaptive immunity are B and T lymphocytes. The **B lymphocyte**, the main actor of humoral immunity, produces antibodies. **T lymphocytes**, the key cells in cell-mediated immunity, destroy invading microorganisms and also help B cells to produce antibodies.

Humoral Immunity

B cells, in birds, are derived from the Bursa of Fabricius. In humans, they arise in the fetal liver and from pluripotent stem cells in the bone marrow, where they go through several steps of maturation. The mature cells have several surface markers that identify them as B cells. The mature cells enter the blood circulation, where they migrate to the secondary lymphoid tissues: spleen, lymph nodes, and Peyer's patches in the small intestine.

The main job of B cells is to produce specific antibodies to fight against the particular antigens. First, the naïve B cells need to be activated. Such activation takes place after exposure of the B cells to an antigen. The steps in activating these naïve B-lymphocytes are summarized below:

1. **Recognition.** First, the antigen binds to the **B lymphocyte surface receptor (BCR)**. This activates the B lymphocyte. Such activation may need other stimuli such as CD4+ Helper T cells (a class of T cells that helps B cells to produce antibodies). Usually, infectious agents require such stimuli (**T cell-dependent antigen**); other antigens, such as polysaccharides or lipids, do not (**T cell-independent antigen**).

2. **Proliferation.** Then, the lymphocytes proliferate and make identical cells (clones), a process known as **clonal expansion**.

3. **Differentiation.** The cloned cells then differentiate to become either antibody-producing cells (**plasma cells**) or **memory cells**. Plasma cells are non-dividing B cells. They live for a few days to weeks and die. Memory cells on the other hand, may live for years. Memory cells recognize and

respond to subsequent exposures of the particular organism that stimulated their formation. The response to this second exposure is known as the **secondary immune response**. Those cells that do not differentiate end up dying (**apoptosis**).

Antibodies
Antibodies (also known as **immunoglobulins**, or **Ig** for short) are glycoproteins produced by plasma cells in response to **antigens**, which are foreign microbial and non-microbial substances. In an electrophoresis of a normal serum sample, the immunoglobulins form a broad band in the gamma portion of the protein sample. There are 5 different **isotypes** (classes) of immunoglobulins: **IgG**, **IgA**, **IgM**, **IgE**, and **IgD**. The mnemonic **GAMED** helps to remember them. IgA has subtypes IgA1 and IgA2; IgG has subtypes IgG1, IgG2, IgG3, and IgG4. Each Ig has a different molecular weight and function, but they all share a common structural unit (**Fig. 1-8**).

Each Ig molecule resembles a letter Y, with 2 arms and a stem. There is a flexible area between the arm and the stem, known as the **hinge region**. Cleavage of the hinge region by protease enzymes separates the antibody into two arms and a stem. Each arm has an antigen-binding site and is designated as **Fab** (fragment antigen binding); the stem is designated **Fc** (fragment crystallizable). Fragmentation

of an antibody molecule by proteolytic enzymes helps the study and identification of structure and function of antibody fragments. The Ig molecule, also known as **Ig monomer**, has 2 identical sets of polypeptide chains. The larger ones are called **heavy chains (H)**, and the lighter ones are called **light chains (L)**. Each heavy and light chain is connected by a disulfide bond. A disulfide bond also binds the two heavy chains. The amino terminal domain of heavy and light chains, known as the V region, consists of a variable amino acid sequence that differs from one type of antibody to another. The carboxy (COOH) terminal domains consist of Ig regions that are constant (non-variable amino acid sequence). Each heavy chain has one **V region** and 3 or 4 C regions, designated as CH1, CH2, and CH3, or CH4. Each light chain has one V region, designated as VL, and one C region, designated as CL. The light chain domains (VL and CL) and the heavy chain domains (VH, CH1, CH2, CH3) are also known as **Ig domains**. The variable regions of heavy and light chains collectively are called the **antigen-binding site**. Each antibody molecule has two such binding sites.

Molecular Features of Immunoglobulins
Immunoglobulins may exist in 2 forms: **membrane-bound** (on the B cell surface) and **secretory**. All membrane-bound Igs are monomeric (one unit structure: 2 heavy chains, 2 light chains). Secretory Igs are either monomeric (IgE and IgG) or multimeric, where two or more units bind with each other (IgA and IgM). Features of immunoglobulins are summarized in **Fig. 1-9**.

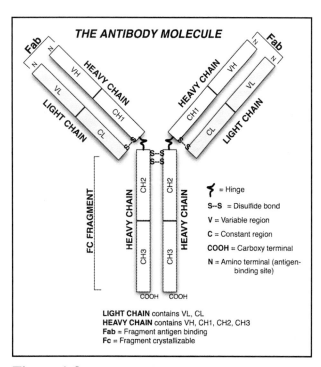

LIGHT CHAIN contains VL, CL
HEAVY CHAIN contains VH, CH1, CH2, CH3
Fab = Fragment antigen binding
Fc = Fragment crystallizable

Figure 1-8

FEATURES OF IMMUNOGLOBULINS		
Immunoglobulin	Structure	Function
IgG	monomer	prominent in secondary response
IgA	dimer (J-chain)	prominent in secretions
IgM	pentamer	prominent in primary antibody response
IgE	long Fc fragment	prominent in worm infestations & allergies. Binds to Fc receptors on mast cells and basophils, causing them to release inflammatory substances
IgD	monomer	receptor on B-lymphocytes

Figure 1-9 (From Goldberg, S., *Clinical Physiology Made Ridiculously Simple*, MedMaster)

- **Immunoglobulin G (IgG)** is a monomer with a molecular weight of 160,000 dalton. It is the most abundant antibody, comprising 75% of total immunoglobulins. With a serum half-life of 23 days, it has the longest life span of the immunoglobulins. It has 4 subclasses: IgG1, IgG2, IgG3, and IgG4, IgG1 being the most abundant and IgG4 the least abundant. IgG1, 2, and 3 participate in complement fixation (a diagnostic test that aids in detection of an antigen, an antibody or both. The complement added to the mixture of an antigen and antibody is consumed [fixed] by the antigen-antibody complex). The clinical significance of IgG4 has not been established. One of the most important features of IgG is its ability to cross the placenta and protect the fetus. It is also involved in Type II hypersensitivity (discussed later) and is prominent in the secondary immune response.
- **Immunoglobulin A (IgA)** has a molecular weight of 170,000 dalton (as a membrane-bound molecule, a monomer) and 350,000 dalton (the secretory form). It comprises 10-15% of the immunoglobulins and has a half-life of 6 days. It is found in bodily secretions: tears, saliva, intestinal mucus, milk, prostatic fluid, and other body secretions. It has 2 subclasses: IgA1 and IgA2. Its main function is mucosal immunity (a system of immunity comprised of lymphoid tissues in mucosal surfaces of the gastrointestinal and respiratory tracts that protects against entrance of bacteria). Both IgA and IgM have a "J chain" (**Fig. 1-9**), a polypeptide chain that joins heavy chains to one another.
- **Immunoglobulin M (IgM)** has the highest molecular weight among the immunoglobulins (900,000 dalton) due to its unique pentamer structure. This is a membrane-bound antigen receptor on the B-cell surface. It is prominent in the primary antibody response.
- **Immunoglobulin E (IgE)** has a long Fc fragment, a molecular weight of 180,000 dalton, and the shortest half-life (2.5 days) among the immunoglobulins. It participates in immediate hypersensitivity (Type I hypersensitivity). This is a type of allergic reaction in which a specific IgE is produced in response to a specific allergen (See Chapter 4). It responds to allergens and parasitic infections by binding to the FcεRI receptor on mast cells and basophils, causing their degranulation and release of mediators of inflammation.
- **Immunoglobulin D (IgD)** is a monomer with a molecular weight of 160,000 dalton and a short half-life of 3 days. It is a membrane-bound antigen receptor on the B–cell surface.

Cell-mediated Immunity

Cell-mediated immunity deals with intracellular bacteria, viruses, and any bacteria that are out of the reach of antibodies. The main players in this type of immunity are T cells. The precursors of T lymphocytes (T cells) arise in the bone marrow. They migrate to the thymus, where they go through several steps of maturation. The main feature of T cell maturation is the expression of surface receptors, known as **T cell receptors (TCR)** and CD4 and CD8 co-receptors. **CD4** and **CD8** co-receptors are T cell surface receptors that bind to peptide (antigen)-MHC complex at the same time as TCR-antigen binding. T helper (CD4+) cells have CD4 co-receptors on their cell surfaces that interact with the peptide-MHC class II complex. T cytotoxic (CD8+) cells have CD8 co-receptors on their cell surface and interact with peptide-MHC class I complex (**Fig. 1-10**). CD4 and CD8 co-receptors participate in signal transduction (transduction of signals from cell surface into the cell to activate T cells).

There are two types of TCR, one with an α and β chain (TCRαβ+, shown in **Fig. 1-11**) and the other with a γ δ chain (TCRγδ+).

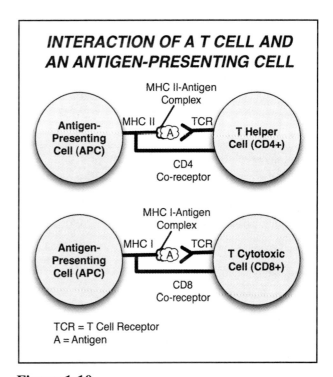

Figure 1-10

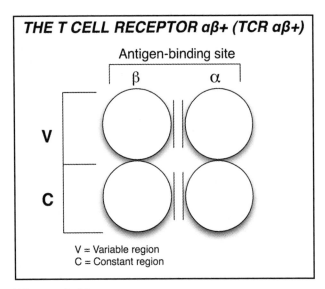

Figure 1-11

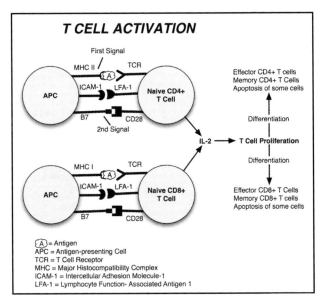

Figure 1-12

The exact functions of TCR γδ+ is unknown. Some TCRαβ+ cells mature to become either CD4+ T cells or CD8+ T cells. The mature cells are then released into the blood circulation. The CD4+ T lymphocytes are also known as T helper lymphocytes (TH); they recognize the MHC class II complex, whereas CD8+ T cells, known as cytolytic or cytotoxic T lymphocytes, recognize the MHC class I complex (discussed later). The mnemonic: **4 x II = 8 x I** helps to remember binding of MHC class I and class II with CD4+ and CD8+ T cells.

T cell activation. Prior to activation, mature T cells are known as naïve T cells. Activation of **naïve cells requires 2 signals (Fig. 1-12).**

The activation of T cells starts by the recognition and binding of TCR to the MHC-antigen complex of antigen-presenting cells (first signal) (**Fig. 1-12**). In addition, the binding of a T cell surface receptor CD28 with B7, a ligand on the antigen-presenting cell (second signal), is also required for the T cell activation. There is also LFA-1 (Lymphocyte Function-Associated Antigen 1), which is found on all T cells, binds to ICAM-1 on antigen-presenting cells and facilitates adhesion of T cells to antigen-presenting cells.

Another factor in this activation is interleukin-2 (IL-2). This cytokine, produced by the naïve T cells, triggers the T cells to divide (**proliferation**). The next step is **differentiation**. Some cells differentiate to **effector cells** (CD4+ T helper cells and CD8+ T-cytolytic cells), while others differentiate to memory cells. Those that do not differentiate eventually die by apoptosis. Effector T cells are differentiated T cells that act to eliminate the antigen. The effector T cells participate in the following functions: **CD4+ T helper cells** produce cytokines that stimulate macrophages for phagocytosis. Other functions of CD4+ T helper cells are summarized in **Fig. 1-13**. **CD8+ T cells** (also known as **cytolytic** or **cytotoxic T cells**) kill virus-infected cells and tumor cells.

Key features of innate and adaptive immunity are summarized in **Fig. 1-14**.

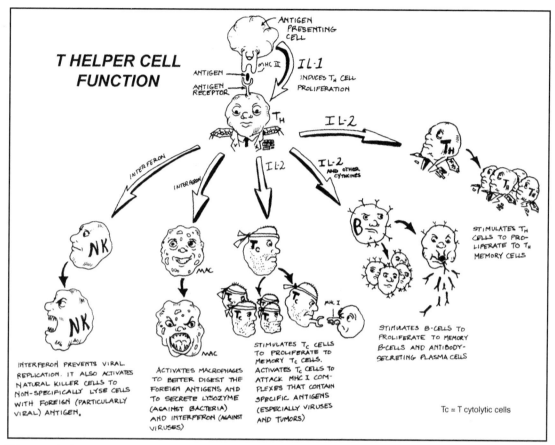

Figure 1-13 (From Goldberg, S., *Clinical Physiology Made Ridiculously Simple*, MedMaster)

FIGURE 1-14

Innate vs. Adaptive Immunity

Immune actions	Innate immunity	Adaptive immunity
Natural antigen barriers (skin, mucous membranes, bodily secretions)	Yes	No
Natural killer (NK) cells (non-specific)	Yes	No
Phagocytosis	Yes	No
Host remembers antigen exposure	No	Yes
Aims at specific antigens	No	Yes
B cells (antibody production) act in the immune response	No	Yes
T cells (cell-mediated immunity) act in the immune response	No	Yes

CHAPTER 2. LYMPHOCYTES AND ANTIGENS

ANTIGEN RECOGNITION

Antigens are molecules recognized by antibodies or T cell receptors. Antibodies can bind to various types of antigenic molecules, e.g., proteins, lipids, nucleic acids, and macro-molecules, such as complex carbohydrates. T cells, on the other hand, only recognize antigens in the form of peptides bound to MHC complex on the surface of host cells. Such antigens either come from the outside environment (**exogenous antigens**) or from host cells (**endogenous antigens**) (**Fig. 2-1**).

Either type of antigen needs to be in peptide form for T cell recognition. The process of converting antigenic protein to peptides is known as **antigen processing**.

Exogenous antigens enter the host cells by a process known as **endocytosis**. In endocytosis the cell membrane invaginates around the antigen and separates from the cell membrane to form a vesicle around the engulfed antigen. The structure containing the antigen is known as an **endosome** (**Fig. 2-1**). The peptides then undergo association with MHC class II and are expressed on the cell surface. This pathway is known as the **endocytic pathway**.

The processing of **endogenous** antigens such as intracellular bacteria (e.g., *Shigella*), viruses, or intracellular parasites (e.g., *Toxoplasma*) takes place in the cytosol.

After entering the host cell, the endogenous antigen undergoes antigen processing. This process involves breakdown of peptides by a complex of proteolytic enzymes known as **proteasomes**. The next step is transportation of peptides to endoplasmic reticulum, where they bind to MHC class I molecules. Finally, the peptide-MHC complex moves to the host cell surface via the Golgi apparatus. This pathway is known as the **cytosolic pathway**. The host cells, also known as **antigen-presenting cells (APC)**, present the peptide-MHC complex to T cells. All nucleated host cells present MHC class I complex and therefore may act as APC. There are only a few types of APCs, however, with an MHC class II complex that presents peptide antigens to T cells. The major APCs of this class are dendritic cells, macrophages, and B cells. APCs with peptide antigen-MHC class II antigen present the antigen–bound complex to CD4+ T cells. APCs with peptide antigen-MHC class I antigen present the antigen-bound complex to CD8+ T cells (**Fig. 2-2**).

MAJOR HISTOCOMPATIBILITY COMPLEX (MHC)

Major Histocompatibility Complex (MHC) is a group of polymorphic genes (various forms of the same gene) located in the short arm of human chromosome 6. MHC, also known as **Human Leukocyte Antigen (HLA) complex**, encodes for two glycoproteins: MHC class I and MHC class II. MHC is also known as Human HLA because of its expression on human leukocytes. Initially identified as important proteins in allograft rejection (allografts are the transplantation of an organ or tissue from a donor to a receiver of the same species), MHC class I and class II have

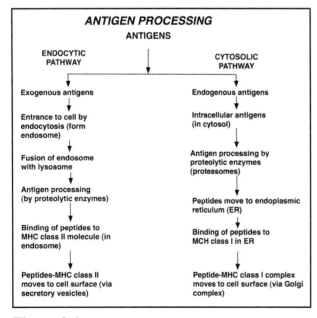

Figure 2-1

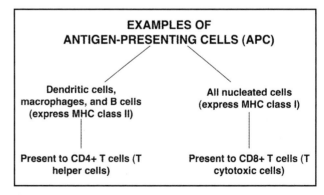

Figure 2-2

another function. They bind to processed antigens (peptides), and after expression on APC surface membranes, present the bound peptides to T cells. The MHC class I and class II molecules differ in amino acid sequences but are similar in three-dimensional structure.

- **MHC class I.** MHC class I consists of two non-covalently bound polypeptide chains: an α (or heavy) chain with molecular weight of 45 kd, and a β2-microglobulin chain with molecular weight of 12 kd. The α chain has 3 subunits designated as α1, α2, and α3 and is anchored to the cell membrane. The α1 and α2 form a cleft for binding of peptides, which is referred to as the **peptide-binding site (Fig. 2-3)**.
- **MHC class II.** MHC class II consists of two polypeptide chains: an α and a β chain. The α chain (molecular weight 33 kd) has 2 subunits, α1 and α2, and is anchored to the cell membrane. The β chain (molecular weight 28 kd) has 2 subunits, β1, and β2, and is also anchored to the cell membrane (**Fig. 2-4**).

Features of MHC class I and II are summarized in **Fig. 2-5**.

MHC POLYMORPHISM

MHC is a polymorphic group of genes. Polymorphism refers to various forms of the same gene within the population. Each variant of the gene is an **allele**. A set of allele variants on a single chromosome is a **haplotype**. Each

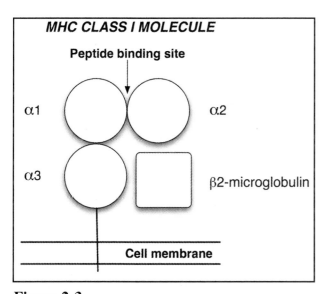

Figure 2-3

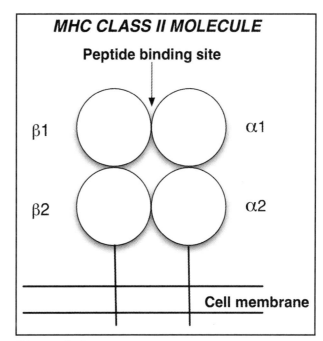

Figure 2-4

individual has multiple copies of MHC class I and class II genes. MHC class I has HLA-A, HLA-B, and HLA-C genes, and MHC class II has HLA-DP, HLA-DQ, and HLA-DR genes. There are also many variations (alleles) of each MHC gene. Therefore, each offspring (who inherits one haplotype from each parent) carries enormous variations of MHC genes. This MHC polymorphism is a useful feature of our defense against antigens, because it makes us well equipped to bind to various forms of antigenic peptides for presentation to T cells (**Fig. 2-5**).

T CELLS AND ANTIGEN-PRESENTING CELL INTERACTION

Interaction of T cells with an antigen-presenting cell (APC) starts with recognition and binding of T cell receptors (TCR) to peptide-MHC complexes on the APC cell surface. As mentioned in Chapter 1, there are two types of TCRs: one type has polypeptide chains α and β, designated as TCR αβ +; the other type has polypeptide chains γ (gamma) and δ (delta), designated as TCR γδ +. The structure of TCR resembles immunoglobulin; each chain (α, β, γ, or δ) consists of a variable domain, designated V, and a constant domain, designated C. The variable region of α and β, or γ and δ forms an **antigen-binding site (Fig. 1-11**, TCR αβ +). TCR is closely associated with 2 other proteins known as **CD3** and ζ (zeta) that

---

FIGURE 2-5

Features of the MCH complex

MHC molecule	Polypeptide chains	Subunits	Anchored to cell membrane	Antigen binding (peptides)	HLA types
MHC class I	α heavy chain (45 kd) β2-microglobulin (12 kd)	α1, α2, α3, β2- microglobulin	α chain	Endogenous antigen	HLA-A HLA-B HLA-C
MHC class II	α (33 kd) β (28 kd)	α1, α2, β1, β2	α and β chains	Exogenous antigen	HLA-DP HLA-DQ HLA-DR

---

participate in **signal transduction** (transduction of signals from the cell surface into the cell to activate T cells). TCR, CD3 and ζ are collectively known as **TCR complex**. There are several other surface receptor proteins known as **accessory molecules** that either participate in signal transduction or adhesion of T cells to APC. They include CD4 and CD8 co-receptors (see Chapter 1 and **Fig. 1-10**), co-stimulatory receptors, and adhesion molecules (**Fig. 2-6**).

FIGURE 2-6

T Cell Receptor and Accessory Molecules

Molecule	Ligand	Functions
TCR	Peptide–MHC	Antigen recognition (first signal for T cell activation)
CD4	MHC class II	Signal transduction
CD8	MHC class I	Signal transduction
CD28	B7	Co-stimulatory signal (second signal for T cell activation)
Adhesion molecules:		
LFA-1	ICAM I, II, III	Adhesion
CD2	LFA-3	
CD44	Hyaluronate	

TCR = T cell receptor
ICAM = Intracellular Adhesion Molecule
LFA = Leukocyte Function Antigen

Costimulatory receptors. Activation and proliferation of T cells depend on two signals. The first signal results from the binding of TCR to the peptide-MHC complex. The second signal results from binding of the **CD28** T cell receptor to B7, an APC surface receptor (**Fig. 1-12**).

Adhesion molecules. Adhesion molecules are a group of T cell surface receptor proteins that bind to their counterpart (**ligand**) on APC. As the name implies, adhesion molecules help (by adhesion) the binding of the T cell receptor to APC. An example of one adhesion molecule (**leukocyte function antigen-1, LFA-1**) and its ligand (**intercellular adhesion molecule-1, ICAM-1**) on APC is demonstrated in **Fig. 1-12**.

ANTIBODY PRODUCTION

Antibody production requires the activation of B cells. As mentioned in Chapter 1, antibody response to an antigen may or may not require the help of T helper cells. Those antigens that are independent of T helper cells are known as **T cell independent antigens** (also known as **thymus-independent antigen**). Those antigens that require the help of T helper cells for an antibody response are known as **T cell dependent antigens** (also known as **thymus-dependent antigen**).

Activation of B Cells

Activation of B cells by **T-cell independent antigen** requires two signals.

The **first signal** arises from binding of B cell receptor (BCR) to the antigenic **epitopes** (epitopes are repeated amino acid sequences throughout the antigen sequence)

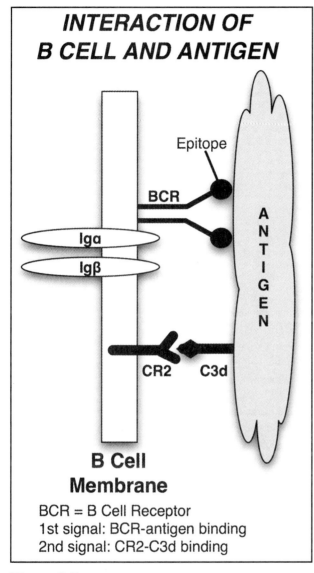

Figure 2-7

Activation of B cells by **T cell dependent antigen** also requires binding of the antigen to BCR. Additionally, the B cell needs to process and present the antigen to CD4 + T cells (T helper cells). See **Fig. 2-8** and section below.

Interaction of B Cells and T Helper Cells

T helper cells recognize the antigen-MHC class II complex and the co-stimulators (B7-1 and B7-2) on the surface of B cells. TCR binds to the antigen-MHC class II complex (first signal for T cell activation). B7-1 and B7-2 bind to CD28 (surface receptor on the T helper cell surface) and stimulate T helper cells (second signal for T cell activation). T helper cells express CD40 ligand, a protein (a cytokine from the tissue necrosis factor family) on their surfaces, which binds to CD40 surface protein on B cells (**Fig. 2-8**). The binding stimulates proliferation and differentiation of B cells. Binding of T helper cells with antigen also stimulates production of several other cytokines (e.g., IL2, IL4, and IL5), which increase B cell proliferation (**Fig. 2-9**). Cytokines will be discussed in Chapter 3.

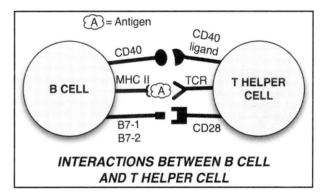

Figure 2-8

(**Fig. 2-7**). The cytoplasmic tail of the BCR is short and therefore unable to transduce the signal into the cell. The BCR has two associated polypeptide chains: Ig α and Ig β. These two have longer cytoplasmic tails and are able to transduce the signal from the cell surface into the cell. After a series of enzymatic events, transcription factors are activated. These factors express genes responsible for B cell activation.

The **second signal** is produced when CR2, a member of the B cell co-receptor complex, binds to an antigen-bound complement C3d. In fact, the antigen-bound complement C3d binds to the CR2 and the BCR at the same time (**Fig. 2-7**).

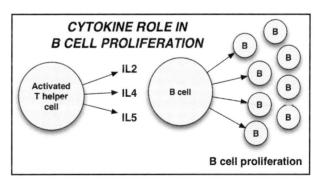

Figure 2-9

Dealing with many antigens requires an efficient system. The immune system confronts thousands of antigens, yet we do not have an antibody molecule for each invading antigen. The good news is that the immune system can rearrange an antibody's structure to deal with many kinds of encountered antigen. Recall the structure of an immunoglobulin (**Fig. 1-8**). Each heavy and light chain has a variable (V) region. The variable regions of heavy and light chains have certain regions (**hypervariable regions**) that are more variable than the rest of the V regions. The remaining amino acid sequences are less variable and are known as **framework** regions. Hypervariable regions are also referred to as **complementarity-determining regions (CDRs)** because they complement the structure of binding antigens (**Fig. 2-10**). Each heavy and light chain has three hypervariable regions. The hypervariable regions of heavy and light chains form antigen-binding sites. Each antibody molecule has two such binding sites. When the body encounters an antigen, our immunoglobulin genes (heavy and light chain variable regions) can rearrange genes to produce an antibody molecule that is specific to the encountered antigen. Therefore, the body could make millions of antibody molecules by just rearranging the immunoglobulin genes (**Fig. 2-10**).

Isotope Switching

Another efficient way to produce antibodies is **isotype switching**. This occurs when activated B cells produce one type of antibody (**isotype**) and, by switching a C region when needed, produce another type of antibody. For example,

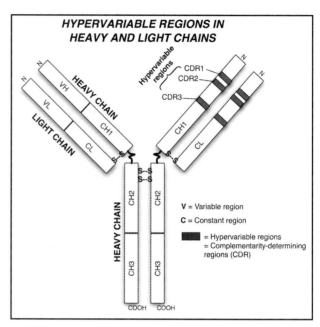

Figure 2-10

when needed, B cells may produce IgE (when exposed to a parasite) and then switch to produce an IgG (when confronting a bacterium).

T cell receptors (TCRs), like BCRs (membrane-bound immunoglobulins), also have variable regions (**Fig. 1-11**). TCRs, like immunoglobulins, can rearrange their variable genes (of α and β chains.) This rearrangement helps, because it allows the TCRs to recognize and bind a variety of antigenic peptide-MHC complexes.

CHAPTER 3.   OTHER IMPORTANT COMPONENTS OF THE IMMUNE SYSTEM

FIGURE 3-1

Eosinophil Features

Feature	Characteristic
Cell type	Granulocyte
Origin	Bone marrow
Size	12-17 μm
Nucleus	Bilobed
Morphologic distinction under light microscope	Stains red due to affinity of MBP granules with eosin dye
Half-life	1-2 days in peripheral blood and several days in tissues
Cytoplasmic contents	Eosinophil cytoplasm carries various granules containing proteins such as MBP, EDN, EPO, ECP, cytokines, chemokinens, and several other mediators
Function	Participates in allergic responses (late phase, a phase Type I hypersensitivity occurring several hours after allergen exposure), and in antiparasitic infection (helminths). It also acts as an antigen-presenting cell.

MBP = Major Basic Protein
EDN = Eosinophil-Derived Neurotoxin
EPO = Eosinophil Peroxidase
ECP = Eosinophil Cationic Protein

EOSINOPHILS

Structure of eosinophils. Eosinophils, like basophils and neutrophils, are granulocytes, cells containing granules, which derive from hematopoetic stem cells. Eosinophils are phagocytic cells that constitute 1-3% of peripheral blood cells. The majority of eosinophils, however, remain in the bone marrow (during maturation) and in various tissues. Eosinophils have numerous granules in their cytoplasm, which contain several types of proteins. One of the main proteins of these granules, **Major Basic Protein (MBP)**, has affinity for **eosin**, an acidic dye that causes the reddish stain of the granules. The protein contents of these granules have

various functions that collectively contribute to the role of eosinophils in allergic immune responses and parasitic infections (discussed below). Other proteins of eosinophil granules include **Eosinophil Peroxidase**, **Charcot-Leyden Crystals**, **lysophosphatase** and a few others (See the next section for discussion of their functions). The nucleus of an eosinophil is bilobed; this and the red stain of the granules give the unique appearance of the eosinophil under a light microscope.

Eosinophil cell membranes carry various receptors for binding IgE, IgG, and complement. Binding of the IgE receptor on the eosinophil to the IgE-antigen complex results in activation of the eosinophils and release of cytoplasmic granules, an action known as **degranulation**. The granular proteins are cytotoxic and damage the invading antigen. The features of eosinophils are summarized in **Fig. 3-1**.

Function of eosinophils. There are two phases of Type I hypersensitivity (Type I allergy): the **early phase** and the **late phase**. Eosinophils participate in the late phase (see Chapter 4).

In addition to the allergic response, eosinophils also fight against parasites, mainly helminths (roundworms).

FIGURE 3-2

Function of Proteins in Eosinophil Granules

Proteins	Function
MBP	• Tissue toxicity • Antiparasitic effect • Used as a marker of eosinophil activity in asthma
ECP	• Tissue toxicity • Antiparasitic effect • Used as a marker of eosinophil activity in asthma • Neurotoxin
EDN	Neurotoxin
EPO	• Tissue toxicity • Antiparasitic effect

MBP = Major Basic Protein
ECP = Eosinophil Cationic Protein
EDN = Eosinophil-Derived Neurotoxin
EPO = Eosinophil Peroxidase

The eosinophil's artillery is the cytotoxic protein contents of its granules, such as MBPs. The function of eosinophil granules is summarized in **Fig. 3-2**. Diseases associated with eosinophils are discussed in Chapter 4.

BASOPHILS

Structure of basophils. Basophils are granulocytes, which derive from hematopoetic stems cells in the bone marrow. Basophils are 5-7 μm in diameter and constitute no more than 1% of nucleated cells in the marrow or peripheral blood. The basophil nucleus, unlike that of eosinophils, is multilobed. When a basophil binds to an IgE-coated antigen, the basophil becomes activated and releases the contents of its secretory granules. The granules release histamine within 5 minutes. Then the basophil releases leukotriene C4 (a lipid mediator produced by a lipoxygenase pathway that causes bronchoconstriction by binding to receptors on smooth muscle cells) within 5-30 minutes. The basophil also releases cytokines TNF-α and IL-4 from minutes to hours after basophil activation. Features of basophils are summarized in **Fig. 3-3**.

Function of basophils. Basophils and mast cells are the main effector cells in the immediate hypersensitivity reaction (See Chapter 4). Mast cells and basophils are similar in many respects. One main similarity is possession of high affinity receptors (known as **FcϵRI**) on their cell surface membranes. This receptor has a high affinity for binding IgE on the surface of the invading allergen. After binding of this high affinity receptor to IgE-coated antigen, the basophils and mast cells are activated and release the contents of their secretory granules. Some of these secretory granules release cytokines IL-4 and TNF-α minutes to hours after allergen exposure and contribute to the inflammatory process. Neutrophils, eosinophils, and TH2 cells also contribute to the inflammatory process. Basophils and mast cells also resemble each other in the similarity of the contents of their mediators. Some examples of the common mediators are illustrated in **Fig. 3-4**.

MAST CELLS

Structure of mast cells. Mast cells originate from the bone marrow stem cells. The undifferentiated mast cells are released into the circulation and differentiate upon arriving at the tissues. These differentiated mast cells measure 10-15 μm in diameter and, like eosinophils and basophils, have secretory granules that carry a variety of proteins. As mentioned earlier, mast cells share several similarities with basophils: the contents of their secretory proteins and the

---

FIGURE 3-3

Features of Basophils

Feature	Characteristic
Cell type	Granulocyte
Origin	Bone marrow
Size	12-15 μm
Nucleus	Multilobed
Distribution	Peripheral blood, tissues
Morphologic distinction under light microscope	Multilobed nucleus, bluish color when stained with the basic dye, methylene blue
Half-life	Days
Cytoplasmic granule contents	Histamine, Major Basic Protein, Charcot-Leyden protein, chondroitin sulfate, neutral proteinases, Leukotriene C4, TNF-α, IL-4
Function	• It is one of the effector cells in immediate hypersensitivity. • It also participates in the late phase reaction.

---

high affinity receptor for IgE, FcϵRI. Mast cells travel through the circulation and reside in the skin and connective tissues as well as the mucosal epithelium of the gastrointestinal, urinary, and respiratory tracts. Features of mast cells are summarized in **Fig. 3-5**.

Function of mast cells. Mast cells are the major effector cells in the immediate hypersensitivity reaction. Binding of the high affinity receptor FcϵRI on their cell surfaces with the IgE-coated allergen results in the activation and release of their secretory granules. The major mediator of mast cells (histamine) causes the known **wheal and flare reaction** (**Fig 3-6**). This reaction is due to vasodilation, vascular leakage, edema (wheal), and redness (flare) in the affected area. In addition to histamines, several other secretory proteins, some unique to mast cells and others similar in both mast cells and basophils, participate in the allergic response (**Fig. 3-4**).

CYTOKINES

Cytokines (cyto = cell; kinesis = movement) are a group of proteins secreted by different cells in the body to help

FIGURE 3-4

Common Mediators in Mast Cells and Basophils

Secretory protein	Type of protein	Functions
Histamine	Vasoactive amines	• Vasodilates, increases vascular permeability • Bronchospasm
Neutral proteases (Tryptase, chymase carboxypeptidase, cathepsin)	Enzyme	• Degrades tissues • Damages microbial structures
Chondroitin Sulfate	Proteoglycan	Participates in structural matrix of granules
Platelet-activating factor	Lipid mediator	• Attracts leukocytes • Increases vascular permeability •Activates neutrophils, eosinophils, and platelets • Bronchoconstricts
Leukotriene C4 (LTC4), D4 (LTD4), and E4 (LTE4)	Lipid mediator	• Bronchospasm • Increases vascular permeability and constriction of arterial, arteriolar, and intestinal smooth muscle
Prostaglandin D2 (PGD2)	Lipid mediator	• Vasodilates • Increases vascular permeability • Bronchoconstricts • Inhibits platelet aggregation • Stimulates neutrophil chemotaxis (attracts neutrophils)
TNF-α	Cytokines	Activates neutrophils
IL-4	Cytokines	• Promotes TH2 differentiation, isotype switching to IgE • B cell proliferation • Eosinophil and mast cell growth and function
IL-5	Cytokines	• Stimulates eosinophil production, activation, growth, and differentiation • Stimulates B lymphocyte proliferation
IL-6	Cytokines	Induces fever, acute phase response (liver)
IL-13	Cytokines	Similar to IL-4

FIGURE 3-5

Features of Mast Cells

Feature	Characteristic
Origin	Bone marrow
Size	10-15 μm
Nucleus	Bilobed or multilobed
Distribution	Skin and connective tissues
Morphologic distinction under light microscope	Purplish color due to stained granules
Half-life	Weeks to months
Examples of cytoplasmic granules contents	Histamine, heparin chondroitin sulfate, proteases
Function	• It is one of the main effector cells in immediate hypersensitivity. • It produces wheal and flare by releasing histamine.

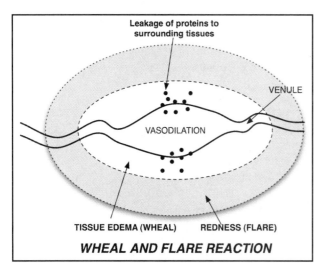

Figure 3-6

cell-to-cell communication and inflammatory and immune response reactions. Traditionally, these proteins were named **lymphokines**, when secreted from lymphocytes, and **monokines**, when secreted from monocytes and macrophages. Studies have shown that lymphokines are products of other cells besides lymphocytes; likewise, besides monocytes and macrophages, other cells produce monokines. Therefore, cytokines is a more appropriate term for these proteins.

Secretion of cytokines starts with stimulation of the cytokine-producing cell (e.g., T helper cell) by an antigen. The secreted cytokines (e.g., IL-4) then bind to receptors on the surface membrane of the target cells (e.g., B cell) and activate them to perform their biological functions (e.g., B cell proliferation) (**Fig. 3-7**).

Sites of cytokine action. Cytokines exert their action locally or systemically. Cytokines may bind to the cytokine receptors on the surface membranes of the same cells that secreted them. This action of cytokines is known as **autocrine action** (**Fig. 3-8A**).

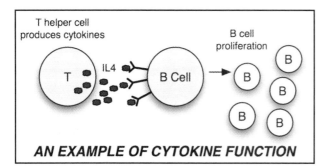

Figure 3-7

Paracrine action occurs when cytokines act locally on the neighborhood cells (**Fig. 3-8B**).

Endocrine action occurs when cytokines act on cells distant from their production site (**Fig. 3-8C**).

Function of cytokines. Cytokines are **pleiotropic**. That is, they exert multiple effects on various cell types. Cytokines may have **synergistic**, **antagonistic**, or **redundancy** effects. A **synergistic** effect occurs when different cytokines show additive effects; i.e., the combined effects of cytokines are more than the effects of a single one. An **antagonistic** effect occurs when two or more cytokines antagonize each other's effects. **Redundancy** is two or more cytokines eliciting the same function without adding to one another's effect.

Classification of Cytokines

Cytokines are classified into **interleukins (IL)**, **interferons (IFN)**, **Tumor Necrosis Factor (TNF)**, **chemokines**, and **Colony Stimulating Factors (CSF)** (**Fig. 3-9**).

- **Interleukins (IL)** are so named because they originate from leukocytes. They are numbered based on the sequence of their discovery. There are at least 30 interleukins, and the numbers may increase as we learn more about cell-cell interactions. Each

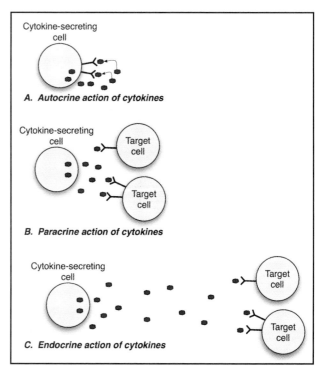

Figure 3-8

FIGURE 3-9

Classification of Cytokines

Type	Source	Function
Interleukin (IL)	Leukocytes	• E.g., IL-2 causes stimulation and proliferation of T cells, B cells and Natural Killer (NK) cells
Interferon (IFN)	• Lymphocytes, dendritic cells, macrophages (IFN-α) • Fibroblasts (IFN-β) • Natural Killer (NK) cells, T cells and other cells (IFN-γ)	• Antiviral activity, expression of MHC class I, activates NK cells (IFN-α, IFN-β) • Activation of macrophages, expression of MHC class I and II, increases antigen presentation (IFN-γ)
Tumor Necrosis Factor (TNF)	Macrophages and other cells	• Induction of fever • Production of acute phase proteins • Apoptosis • Septic shock
Chemokines	Various cells	Regulate chemotaxis
Colony Stimulating Factor (CSF)	• Bone marrow stem cells • T cells • Other cells	• Stimulate the progenitor cells to differentiate into granulocytes, monocytes, and erythrocytes

interleukin has its own function. For example, IL-2, secreted from T cells, stimulates proliferation and differentiation of T cells, B cells, and Natural Killer cells. IL-1, secreted from a variety of cells such as monocytes, macrophages, T, B and NK cells, induces fever and stimulates neutrophil production, among other functions.

• **Interferons (IFN)** are cytokines produced by lymphocytes, dendritic cells, macrophages (**IFN-α**, also known as leukocyte interferon), fibroblasts (**IFN-β**, also known as fibroblast interferon), NK cells, T cells and other cells (**IFN-γ**, also known as immune interferon). The main functions of interferon are antiviral activity (mainly IFN-α and IFN-β), expression of class I MHC (IFN-α and IFN-β), activation of macrophages, expression of both MHC class I and II (IFN-γ), and increasing antigen presentation (IFN-γ) (**Fig. 3-10**).

• **Tumor Necrosis Factor (TNF)** is a cytokine produced by macrophages and other cells in response to gram negative and other microbial infections. The name originates from the observation that the cytokine caused tumor necrosis in animals. This cytokine was also independently isolated and identified as a cause of **cachexia** (wasting disease) in cows and was named **cachectin**. Further investigation revealed that the two components

(TNF and cachectin) are in fact the same protein (TNF). Tumor necrosis factor has various functions in our immune system. One of its systemic effects is induction of fever by stimulating the hypothalamus. It also stimulates the liver to produce **acute phase proteins**. These are proteins produced in the liver and secreted into the blood after infection. Other functions of TNF include the induction of **apoptosis** (programmed cell death) and septic shock.

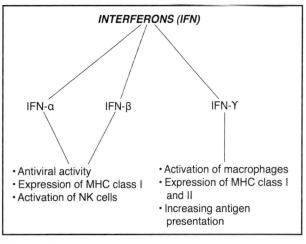

Figure 3-10

FIGURE 3-11

Examples of Diseases Treated with Cytokines

Medication: Generic (Brand name)	Cytokine	Class or type	Treatment indication
Anakinra (Kineret)	IL-1	IL-1 receptor antagonist	Rheumatoid arthritis
Oprelvekin (Neumega)	IL-11	Interleukin	Prevention of severe thrombocytopenia
Roferon	Interferon alpha-2a	Interferon	Chronic hepatitis C, hairy cell leukemia, chronic myelogenous leukemia
Interferon alpha-2b (Intron A)	Interferon alpha-2b	Interferon	Hairy cell leukemia, malignant melanoma, follicular lymphoma, condylomata acuminata, AIDS-related Kaposi sarcoma, chronic hepatitis B and C
Interferon beta-la (Rebif)	Interferon beta-la	Interferon	Multiple sclerosis
Interferon beta-lb (Betaseron)	Interferon beta-lb	Interferon	Multiple sclerosis
Interferon gamma-lb (Actimmune)	Interferon gamma	Interferon	Chronic granulomatous disease, osteopetrosis
Etanercept (Enbrel)	A dimeric fusion protein consisting of TNF receptor and Fc portion of human IgG1	TNF receptor	Rheumatoid arthritis, juvenile rheumatoid arthritis, psoriatic arthritis, ankylosing spondylitis, plaque psoriasis
Filgrastim (Neupogen)	Granulocyte colony stimulating factor (G-CSF)	Colony-stimulating factor	• Stimulated production of neutrophils • Reduces infection in cancer patients receiving myelosuppressive chemotherapy • Used in patients with acute myeloid leukemia receiving induction or consolidation chemotherapy • Used in cancer patients receiving bone marrow transplants
Sargramostim (Leukine)	Granulocyte-macrophage colony stimulating factor (GM-CSF)	Colony stimulating factor	Post-chemotherapy in acute myelogenous leukemia, bone marrow transplantation failure
Epotein alpha (Epogen)	Erythopoietin	Hematopoietic cytokine	• Anemia of chronic renal failure • Anemia in cancer patients on chemotherapy

- **Chemokines** (chemoattractant cytokines) are a family of over 50 low molecular weight proteins, secreted by various cells. Chemokines help regulate **chemotaxis**, i.e., movements of cells (leukocytes) from the blood to the tissues (the site of inflammation and injury).
- **Colony-stimulating factors (CSF)** are cytokines produced by bone marrow stem cells, T cells, macrophages, and other cells. They stimulate the progenitor cells to differentiate into granulocytes, monocytes, platelets, and erythrocytes. The type of CSF derives from the name of the cells that they help produce. For example, **Granulocyte Colony Stimulating Factor (G-CSF)** helps the production of neutrophils. It reduces infection in cancer patients receiving myelosuppressive chemotherapy and bone marrow transplants, and in patients with acute myeloid leukemia receiving **induction** or **consolidation chemotherapy**. **Induction chemotherapy** refers to the use of conventional chemotherapy prior to stem cell transplant. **Consolidation chemotherapy** refers to chemotherapy after remission to fight against the remaining cancer cells and help prevent relapse. **Granulocyte-Monocyte Colony Stimulating Factor (GM-CSF)** is used post-chemotherapy in acute myelogenous leukemia and bone marrow transplantation failure.

Cytokines and Disease

Therapeutic use of commercially prepared cytokines has helped thousands of patients with various diseases. Although the use of such products is usually costly and bears the risk of adverse reactions, their use may be the only alternative modality. Some examples of diseases treated with cytokines are summarized in **Fig. 3-11**.

PART II. CLINICAL IMMUNOLOGY

CHAPTER 4. HYPERSENSITIVITY

Hypersensitivity refers to sensitization of the immune system by repeated exposure to an allergen. **Allergens** are exogenous antigens (usually proteins), such as tree pollens and pet danders, that upon inhalation stimulate an immune response known as a **hypersensitivity (allergic) reaction**.

The clinical presentation of hypersensitivity reactions varies according to the underlying mechanism. The traditional (**Gel** and **Coombs**) classifications of hypersensitivity reactions divides **hypersensitivity** reactions into 4 groups: **Types I, II, III,** and **IV** (**Fig. 4-1**).

FIGURE 4-1

Gel and Coombs Classification of Hypersensitivity Reactions

Type of hypersensitivity reaction	Also known as
Type I	Immediate hypersensitivity, anaphylactic, or IgE-mediated
Type II	Antibody (IgG or IgM) mediated
Type III	Immune complex mediated
Type IV	Cell-mediated or delayed type

TYPE I HYPERSENSITIVITY REACTION (IgE-MEDIATED)

Type I hypersensitivity reaction is an immediate IgE-mediated immune response to an allergen (after repeated exposure to the allergen). Individuals who develop this type of reaction have a genetic predisposition (**atopic**) and are sensitized by repeated exposure to a specific type of an allergen. The mast cells in such individuals become sensitized, and upon subsequent exposure, degranulate and release various secretory granules, resulting in a localized or systemic immune reaction. Type I hypersensitivity reaction

consists of an early phase and a late phase immune response. The early phase of an allergic reaction occurs within minutes of an allergen exposure. This is a result of histamine release from mast cells, which causes vasodilation, edema, and congestion. The late phase of an allergic reaction occurs 2 to 24 hours after the allergen exposure. This is an inflammatory process in which eosinophils, neutrophils, and T cells infiltrate the area.

The mechanism of the Type I hypersensitivity reaction involves a multistep process (**Fig. 4-2**). It starts with the exposure of the host to an allergen. The TH2 helper cells get activated.

There are two types of T helper cells: TH1 and TH2. The TH2 is involved in Type I hypersensitivity (TH1 is involved in Type IV allergy, discussed below). The activation of TH2 and the binding to the B cells stimulates the B cells to undergo class switching; that is, the B cells that are capable of producing IgG and IgM, upon stimulation by TH2 cells, switch to produce IgE antibody. The B cells produce a specific IgE to the exposed allergen. Shortly thereafter, the IgE binds to high affinity receptor FcεRI on the surface of the mast cells. At this time, the mast cells are sensitized; this means that upon exposure to the same allergen, the mast cells degranulate and release their contents. The contents of the mast cells, as discussed before, include various mediators. The major mediator, histamine, causes vasodilation, vascular leakage, and edema.

Some examples of Type I hypersensitivity diseases are outlined in **Fig. 4-3**. The prototype of this category, allergic rhinitis, is briefly discussed below.

Allergic Rhinitis

Allergic rhinitis is a Type I hypersensitivity disease that causes seasonal or perennial (year-round) symptoms in susceptible individuals. The disease causes various nasal and upper respiratory symptoms. Although **rhinitis** means an inflammation (itis) of the nose (rhino), allergic rhinitis refers to the combination of symptoms that also affect the ears, pharynx, oral cavity, bronchial tree, and, occasionally, the eyes. The term **rhinoconjunctivitis** refers to the combined symptoms of allergic rhinitis and allergic reaction in the eyes (conjunctivitis). The eye symptoms include erythema, watery eyes, and pruritus (**Fig. 4-4**).

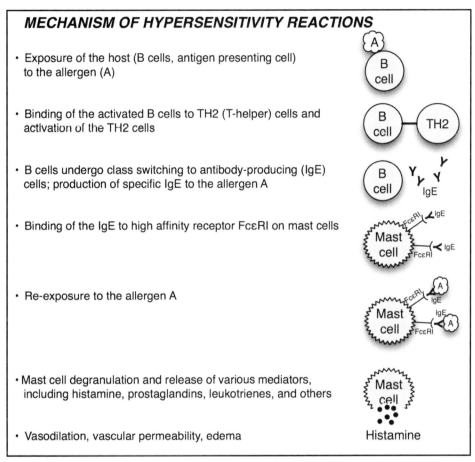

MECHANISM OF HYPERSENSITIVITY REACTIONS

• Exposure of the host (B cells, antigen presenting cell) to the allergen (A)

• Binding of the activated B cells to TH2 (T-helper) cells and activation of the TH2 cells

• B cells undergo class switching to antibody-producing (IgE) cells; production of specific IgE to the allergen A

• Binding of the IgE to high affinity receptor FcεRI on mast cells

• Re-exposure to the allergen A

• Mast cell degranulation and release of various mediators, including histamine, prostaglandins, leukotrienes, and others

• Vasodilation, vascular permeability, edema

Figure 4-2

The symptoms of allergic rhinitis are due to mediators released by mast cells, histamine being the main cause of symptoms. In order to elicit symptoms, histamine needs to bind to histamine receptors. There are 4 types of histamine receptors : H1, H2, H3, and H4. In allergic rhinitis, the H1 receptors are the main target of histamine interaction. H1 receptors are distributed in various tissues, such as the nasal passages, oral cavity, conjunctiva, bronchi, and small intestine. Binding of histamine to H1 receptors causes dilation of blood vessels, resulting in capillary permeability and contraction of smooth muscle (small intestine and bronchi, involved in anaphylaxis). The blockage of H1 receptors is an important intervention in allergic rhinitis and allergic rhinoconjunctivitis symptoms.

Two kinds of allergens cause allergic rhinitis: indoor and outdoor. Indoor allergens include dust mites (microscopic eight-legged organisms that feed on organic matter, such as feathers and human skin scales), molds, cockroaches, and pet danders. Outdoor allergens include insects (bees, yellow jackets, wasps) and pollens (trees, grasses and weeds). Some examples of indoor and outdoor allergens are outlined in **Fig. 4-5**.

Management of allergic rhinitis. The management of allergic rhinitis includes:

1. Precaution and control measures (**Fig. 4-6**)
2. Medications (**Fig. 4-7**)
3. Allergy vaccination (immunotherapy)

Medications to control allergic rhinitis and allergic rhinoconjunctivitis include antihistamines, mast cell stabilizers, and antileukotrienes. Various forms of drug delivery of antihistamines include nasal sprays, eye drops, and creams (for pruritus due to Type I hypersensitivities such as bee stings). These medications, their

---

FIGURE 4-3

Examples of Type I Hypersensitivity Diseases

Disease	Common symptoms
Allergic rhinitis	Nasal congestion, rhinorrhea (runny nose), postnasal drip, sneezing, pruritus (oral and nasal mucosa)
Allergic rhinoconjunctivitis	Allergic rhinitis symptoms plus itchy, watery, and red eyes
Allergic asthma	Shortness of breath, chest tightness, wheezing, cough
Food allergy	Skin symptoms: urticaria (hives), angioedema (swelling of blood vessel wall), anaphylaxis (in extreme form)
Bee sting allergy	As in food allergy. In extreme form: anaphylaxis
Occupational allergy	Depending on the area of body exposure: respiratory (like allergic asthma); skin (urticaria, angioedema)
Anaphylaxis (the ultimate form of Type 1 hypersensitivity reaction)	Symptoms of cardiovascular collapse: hypotension, tachycardia, asphyxia Skin symptoms: generalized urticaria; angioedema, including laryngoedema (edema of larynx); edema of smooth muscles in gastrointestinal mucosa, causing abdominal pain

---

FIGURE 4-4

Symptoms of Allergic Rhinitis and Allergic Rhinoconjunctivitis

Anatomical site	Symptoms
Eyes	Red, watery, itchy
Nose	Nasal congestion, blocked nose, rhinorrhea (watery nose), itching (mucosa)
Oral cavity	Postnasal drip, itchy oral mucosa (especially palate), sneezing
Ears	Plugged ears

FIGURE 4-5

Indoor and Outdoor Allergens that Cause Allergic Rhinitis

Type of allergen	Type of environment	Examples
Pollens	Outdoor	Trees, grasses, weeds
Insects	Outdoor	Bees, yellow jackets, wasps
Insects	Indoor	Cockroaches
Molds	Indoor (originated from outdoor by getting into indoor environment from an open door or a window)	*Aspergillus, Penicillium*
Dust mites	Indoor	House dust mites
Pets (hair, danders)	Indoor	Cats, dogs
Pets (urine)	Indoor	Rodents

mechanisms, and several examples of each are summarized in **Fig. 4-7**.

Allergy vaccination, also known as **allergy immunotherapy**, is the gradual administration of a specific allergen to an individual to produce immunity against future exposure to the same allergen (See Chapter 8).

FIGURE 4-6

**Precautions and Control Measures
for Allergic Rhinitis**

**Examples of precautions and
control measures**

Outdoor allergens

| Trees, grasses, weeds | • Avoid direct exposure.
• Do not mow the lawn. If you do, wear a mask. |
| Insects | • Do not wear colorful shirts.
• Avoid using perfumes and scented cosmetics.
• Use protective clothing (long sleeves).
• Dispose of trash and cover the trash containers. |

Indoor allergens

Dust mites	• Avoid carpets; dust mites accumulate there. • Use dust mite proof encasing for beddings. • Decrease indoor humidity to below 55%. • Do not play with stuffed animal toys (children). • Do not use upholstered furniture.
Pets	• Do not keep indoor pet if allergic. • Keep pet out of bedroom.
Cockroaches	• Dispose of food remains in closed door trash containers. • Keep indoor humidity below 55%.
Molds	• Clean visible molds with bleach. • Keep indoor humidity below 55%. • Fix leaky plumbing to prevent a damp environment.

FIGURE 4-7

Classes of Medications for Allergic Rhinitis

Medication class	Mechanism	Examples
Antihistamines	Blocks H1 receptors	Oral (loratadine, fexofenadine, cetirizine) Ophthalmic (olopatadine[1]) Nasal spray (azelastine)
Mast cell stabilizer	Prevents mast cells from degranulation	Nasal (chromolyn sodium) Ophthalmic (olopatadine[1])
Nasal steroids	Anti-inflammatory	fluticasone, mometazone
Antileukotrienes	Leukotriene receptor antagonist	monteleukast, zafirleukast
Antileukotrienes	Lipooxygenase inhibitor	zileuton

(1) Antihistamine with mast cell stabilizing effect

2. **Antibody-dependent cellular cytotoxicity (ADCC).** An IgG binds to the surface antigen on an infected cell. The NK cells recognize and kill the antibody-coated infected cell (**Fig. 4-9**).
3. **Complement activation.** The binding of an IgG to an antigen can activate the complement system and cause the lysis of the antigen by the membrane attack complex (**MAC**) or by phagocytosis (**Fig. 1-7**).

TYPE II HYPERSENSITIVITY REACTION (ANTIBODY-MEDIATED)

Type II hypersensitivity reactions (also known as **antibody-mediated**) involve the interaction of a non-IgE antibody (IgG or IgM) with a cell surface or an extracellular matrix antigen, which destroys the antigen in one of the following ways:

1. **Opsonization and phagocytosis.** The antibody binds to the antigen and makes it a target for phagocytosis, a process known as **opsonization** (**Fig. 4-8**).

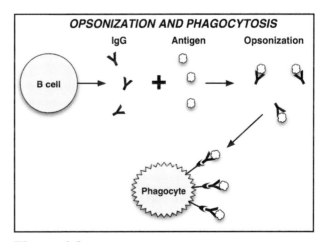

Figure 4-8

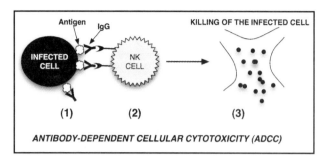

Figure 4-9

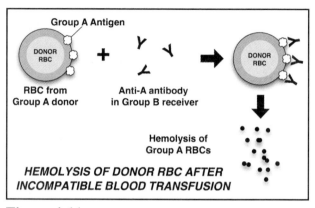

Figure 4-11

Fig. 4-10 summarizes several Type II hypersensitivity diseases. Blood transfusion reaction is briefly discussed below.

Blood Transfusion Reaction

A **blood transfusion reaction** is a host immune response due to a mismatch of the major red blood cell antigens, known as **ABO groups**. An incompatible blood group antigen leads to hemolysis of the donor's red blood cells (**Fig. 4-11**).

The ABO blood group refers to surface membrane markers on various cells, including red blood cells, and dictates the compatibility of a blood transfusion. The ABO blood groups include the following members:

- **Group A.** Group A has two genotypes: AA and AO. Individuals with blood group A have antigen A and anti-B antibody. Group A donors can safely donate blood to group A and receive blood from group A and group O.
- **Group B.** Group B has two genotypes: BB and BO. Individuals with blood group B have antigen

B and anti-A antibody. The group B donors can safely donate blood to group B and receive blood from group B and group O.

- **Group AB.** Group AB has one genotype: AB. Individuals with blood group AB have antigens A and B and no antibody. Therefore, they can donate blood safely to group AB and can receive blood from any group. As a result, they are known as **universal receivers**.
- **Group O.** Group O has one genotype: OO. Individuals with group O have anti-A and anti-B antibodies but no antigen. Therefore, they can donate blood to any group but can only receive blood from group O donors. They are called **universal donors** (**Fig. 4-12**).

TYPE III HYPERSENSITIVITY REACTION (IMMUNE COMPLEX-MEDIATED)

In **Type III hypersensitivity**, the interaction of an antigen and an antibody forms an **immune complex**. This complex usually activates the complement system and is removed by phagocytosis.

The smaller complexes escape phagocytosis and precipitate in blood vessel walls (causing vasculitis), kidney glomeruli (causing nephritis), and synovial membranes (causing arthritis) (**Fig. 4-13**).

Fig. 4-14 lists a number of Type III hypersensitivity diseases. The prototype of Type III hypersensitivity, **serum sickness**, is briefly discussed below.

Serum Sickness

The history of serum sickness goes back to the early 1900s in the treatment for diphtheria. Then, the preparation of diphtheria antitoxin consisted of injecting diphtheria toxin

---

FIGURE 4-10

Examples of Type II Hypersensitivity Reactions

Disease	Involved Antigens
Transfusion reaction	ABO blood group
Autoimmune hemolytic anemia	Rhesus (Rh) blood groups
Autoimmune thrombocytic purpura	Platelet surface membrane proteins
Graves disease	Thyroid stimulating hormone (TSH) receptor
Myasthenia gravis	Acetylcholine receptor

FIGURE 4-12

ABO Blood Groups

Blood group	Genotype	Antigen	Antibody	Safe to donate to	Safe to receive from
A	AA, AO	A	Anti-B	A	A, O
B	BB, BO	B	Anti-A	B	B, O
AB	AB	A and B	No antibody	AB	A, B, AB, O
O	OO	None	Anti-A, anti-B	A, B, AB, O	O

---

into a horse and harvesting the serum after a period of time. The individuals with diphtheria who received such sera developed **serum sickness** 4-21 (usually 8-10) days after serum exposure (**Fig. 4-15**), consisting of fever, lymphadenopathy, urticaria, and other symptoms (**Fig. 4-16**). The symptoms of serum sickness coincided with the formation and precipitation of immune complexes in the tissues. Now that serum diphtheria antitoxin is no longer prepared in horses, other antigens, such as certain medications and anti-sera, cause serum sickness.

Management of serum sickness. Early detection of the offending agent is the key to the successful diagnosis and management of serum sickness. The next step is symptomatic relief of the symptoms. Anti-inflammatory drugs such as nonsteroidal anti-inflammatory drugs (for milder reactions), steroidal anti-inflammatory drugs (for more pronounced reactions), and antihistamines may help the recovery of affected individuals, who usually recover without complications.

TYPE IV HYPERSENSITIVITY REACTION (CELL-MEDIATED; DELAYED TYPE)

Type IV hypersensitivity is an immune reaction in which the T effector cells, CD4+ T helper and CD8+ T cells, are activated by antigens (presented by antigen-presenting cells). The T cells then release cytokines (e.g., IFN-γ), causing activation of phagocytes, leading to tissue inflammation and injury (**Fig. 4-17**). CD8+ cytotoxic T lymphocytes can also kill the infected target cell directly (**Fig. 4-18**).

Mantoux Reaction

The classic example of a cell-mediated immunity reaction is the **Mantoux reaction**. This is an immune allergic contact

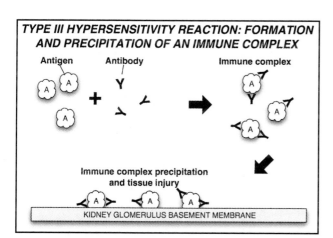

TYPE III HYPERSENSITIVITY REACTION: FORMATION AND PRECIPITATION OF AN IMMUNE COMPLEX

Antigen   Antibody   Immune complex

Immune complex precipitation and tissue injury

KIDNEY GLOMERULUS BASEMENT MEMBRANE

Figure 4-13

FIGURE 4-14

Examples of Type III Hypersensitivity Diseases

Disease	Site of involvement
Serum sickness	Kidneys, joints, blood vessels
Systemic Lupus Erythematosus (SLE)	Kidneys, joints, blood vessels
Post-streptococcal glomerulonephritis	Kidney
Hepatitis	Liver
Rheumatoid arthritis	Joints
Farmer's lung	Lungs

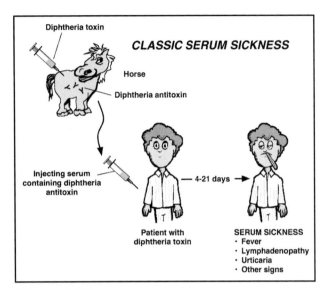

Figure 4-15

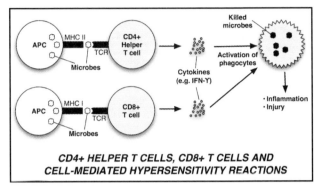

Figure 4-17

dermatitis reaction in sensitized individuals to *Mycobacterium tuberculosis* after a tuberculin test. Injection of tuberculin, a protein extract of *Mycobacterium tuberculosis,* into the skin results in a reaction consisting of redness and a raised, indurated (hardened) area at the site of injection about 48 hours after administration of this antigen.

Allergic Contact Dermatitis

Another example of Type IV hypersensitivity is **allergic contact dermatitis**. This is a cell-mediated hypersensitivity reaction that occurs after contact with various plants (poison ivy), chemicals used in cosmetics, medications (topical antibiotics, anesthetics), jewelry, cleaning products, and industrial reagents (**Fig. 4-19**).

The diagnosis of allergic contact dermatitis includes a history of contact with the suspected allergen and **patch**

testing, as follows. The allergen, embedded on a polyester patch, is placed on the upper back of the affected individual. The patch is removed after 48 hours for preliminary observation and reevaluated 2 days later (see Chapter 6).

Management of allergic contact dermatitis. Management of allergic contact dermatitis includes the avoidance of the offending agent. Antihistamines help the pruritus, and topical intermediate potency corticosteroids such as triamcinolone acetonide 0.1% applied to the affected area (except the face, due to a higher chance of skin atrophy, acne, stretch marks, and other skin side effects) help to alleviate the irritation and inflammation. Patients with severe manifestations of poison ivy or other forms of allergic contact dermatitis can benefit from tapering doses of oral corticosteroids.

EOSINOPHILS AND DISEASE

It is important to introduce other diseases associated with eosinophils and mast cells in this chapter although they are not necessarily part of the hypersensitivity diseases.

Eosinophilia

Eosinophilia refers to an abnormal increase of eosinophils in peripheral blood or tissues. Eosinophilia comes in two categories: **familial** and **acquired**. Familial eosinophilia is a

---

FIGURE 4-16

Symptoms of Serum Sickness

Affected area	Examples
General	Malaise, weakness, fever
Skin	Urticaria, angioedema, rash (vasculitis)
Joints	Arthralgia
Lymph nodes	Lymphadenopathy
Kidney	Glomerulonephritis

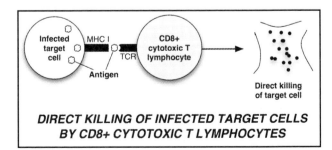

Figure 4-18

FIGURE 4-19

Examples of Allergens that Cause Allergic Contact Dermatitis

Products	Examples of the antigen
Cosmetics	Thimerosal, quaternium, epoxy resin
Jewelry	Nickel
Antibiotics	Neomycin sulfate, benzocaine
Topical medications	Wool (lanolin) alcohols, cinnamic alcohol
Perfumes	Balsam of Peru

FIGURE 4-20

Etiology of Acquired Eosinophilia

Etiology	Examples
Primary	
• Clonal	• Acute leukemia
• Idiopathic	• Hypereosinophilic syndrome
Secondary	
• Infections	• Bacterial, viral, fungal, and parasitic infections
• Fungal	• Allergic bronchopulmonary aspergillosis (ABPA)
• Viral	• Human immunodeficiency virus (HIV), West Nile Virus
• Parasitic	• Ascariasis, Filariasis, Trichinosis
• Medications	• Antibiotics: Penicillin, ampicillin, sulfonamides, minocycline; NSAIDS (non-steroidal anti-inflammatory drugs): aspirin, naproxen, ibuprofen; Antidepressants: trazodone, fluoxetin; Hypoglycemic agents: chlorpropramide
• Allergic diseases	• Allergic rhinitis, asthma
• Malignancies	• Lymphoma

rare autosomal disorder of low clinical significance. Acquired eosinophilia is divided into **primary eosinophilia** and **secondary eosinophilia**. **Primary eosinophilia** subdivides into **clonal eosinophilia**, where there is cytogenetic or histologic evidence of myeloid malignancy (e.g., acute myeloid leukemia), and **idiopathic**, where the etiology is unknown. **Secondary eosinophilia** is due to parasitic infection, medications, or other causes. Various causes of acquired eosinophilias and some examples of each are summarized in **Fig. 4-20**.

Eosinophils can infiltrate various organs and cause damage by releasing the contents of their toxic granules. Examples of affected organ systems and associated diseases are summarized in **Fig. 4-21**.

Hypereosinophilic syndrome (HES), an example of primary eosinophilia, is discussed below. **Allergic rhinitis**, an example of secondary eosinophilia, is discussed earlier in this chapter.

Hypereosinophilic syndrome (HES; also known as **hypereosinophilic syndromes)** is a heterogeneous group of diseases with the following diagnostic criteria:

1. Presence of peripheral eosinophilia with absolute eosinophil counts of 1500 cells/μL or greater for at least 6 months.
2. Absence of an identifiable etiology of eosinophilia.
3. Evidence of organ involvement (eosinophil infiltration).

The majority of individuals affected by HES are men (male: female 9:1) in the 20-50 years range, although the disease can affect other ages as well. The clinical features of the disease depend on which organ is involved. Some reported symptoms include shortness of breath, cough, weakness, fever, myalgia, angioedema, rash, and blurry vision.

FIGURE 4-21

Organ Systems Affected by Eosinophilia

Organ system	Disease
Hematic	Mastocytosis
Pulmonary	Eosinophilic pneumonia (primary or idiopathic, simple, acute, and chronic), asthma, Allergic Bronchopulmonary Aspergillosis (ABPA)
Cardiac	Hypersensitivity myocarditis
Skin	Atopic dermatitis, chronic urticaria
Gastrointestinal	Eosinophilic gastroenteritis
Immune	Scleroderma, vasculitis (Churg-Straus syndrome, Wegener granulomatosis)

Treatment of HES includes the use of prednisone (anti-inflammatory drug), interferon-α (a cytokine with antiviral effect), and immunosuppressive drugs such as cyclosporin for those refractory to prednisone. The second line of therapy is **imatinib** (a kinase inhibitor) and, finally, patients refractory to medication may benefit from bone marrow transplantation.

MAST CELLS AND DISEASE

Mast cells are major effector cells in immediate Type I hypersensitivity reactions. This chapter presents several examples of diseases in this category. In addition to Type I hypersensitivity reactions, abnormal aggregation of mast cells in tissues causes a disease called **mastocytosis**.

Mastocytosis

Mastocytosis is due to the abnormal aggregation of mast cells in skin, bone marrow, liver, and spleen. Other tissues, however, may also be affected. Stimulation of the vast number of mast cells releases a large amount of histamine, leading to a spectrum of symptoms that include flushing, pruritus, nausea, vomiting, abdominal pain, and, occasionally **anaphylaxis** (a severe form of an allergic reaction in which mast cells and basophil activation and degranulation cause respiratory and cardiovascular collapse). Mastocytosis may be limited to the skin (**cutaneous mastocytosis**). A tan-reddish-brown macule (a flat-surface rash) or a papule (a raised-surface rash) known as **urticaria pigmentosa** is the most common skin manifestation of cutaneous mastocytosis.

FIGURE 4-22

Organ Involvement and Related Symptoms in Systemic Mastocytosis

Organ system	Symptoms
Blood	Flushing
Skin	Pruritus, urticaria
Gastrointestinal tract	Abdominal pain, gastric hypersecretion, nausea, vomiting, diarrhea
Cardiovascular, pulmonary, skin	Anaphylaxis

Aggregation of mast cells in multiple organs, with or without skin involvement, is referred to as **systemic mastocytosis**. Cutaneous mastocytosis usually develops in early childhood while systemic mastocytosis occurs in adults. Examples of the involved organs in systemic mastocytosis and their related symptoms are summarized in **Fig. 4-22**.

Diagnosis of mastocytosis. Diagnosis of mastocytosis includes the history of related symptoms, physical examination with special attention to the skin findings, and diagnostic procedures. The skin lesion (urticaria pigmentosa) requires a biopsy, which shows aggregation of mast cells. The next step is bone marrow aspiration, which reveals aggregates of spindle-shaped mast cells in perivascular, peritrabecular, or intertrabecular locations. Release of histamine can be traced by measuring histamine or histamine metabolites in a 24-hour urine sample. Diagnostic work-up is summarized in **Fig. 4-23**.

FIGURE 4-23

Diagnostic Workup in Mastocytosis

Workup	Procedure	Findings
Examination of the skin	Biopsy of the skin lesions (urticaria pigmentosa)	Mast cell aggregates
Investigation of bone marrow involvement	Bone marrow aspiration	Aggregates of spindle-shaped mast cells in perivascular, peritrabecular, or intertrabecular locations
Tracking histamine release by searching for histamine or metabolites in urine	24-hour urine collection	Increased urine histamine, methylhistamine, methylimidazole acetic acid, and prostaglandin D_2
Blood	Detection of serum tryptase (a neutral protease secreted by the activated mast cells)	Increased serum tryptase

---

Management of mastocytosis. Control of symptoms is the mainstay of the management of mastocytosis. Control of the skin symptoms includes the use of antihistamines for pruritus, photochemotherapy (with psoralen and ultraviolet A, PUVA) for urticaria pigmentosa, and, finally, corticosteroids for the skin lesions. The use of disodium cromoglycate (a mast cell stabilizing compound) is beneficial in managing the gastrointestinal symptoms. Aspirin is useful for flushing because it reduces the effect of prostaglandin D_2 (**Fig. 4-24**).

FIGURE 4-24

Management of Systemic Mastocytosis

Organ system	Condition	Management
Skin	Pruritus	Antihistamines
Skin	Urticaria pigmentosa	Psoralene with ultraviolet light A (PUVA)
Skin	Severe urticaria pigmentosa	Corticosteroids
Gastrointestinal tract	Abdominal pain, diarrhea	Disodium chromoglycate (a mast cell stabilizer)
Gastrointestinal tract	Gastric acid hypersecretion	H2 histamine receptor blocker, proton pump inhibitor
Blood	Flushing	Antihistamine, aspirin

CHAPTER 5.   AUTOIMMUNITY

Soldiers have one main goal: defending their land and citizens. They fight the enemy, not their fellow soldiers. They differentiate the members of their own team from those of the enemy. How? Some differences include the uniforms, the type of weapons, and the combat strategies. Our immune system, like the soldiers, can differentiate our "self-antigens" from "non-self" antigens. In order to stay healthy, it is important that our immune system fight invading organisms and not "self." This is known as **self-tolerance**. Consider self-tolerance a system that keeps the defensive B and T lymphocytes in check to avoid attacking self-antigens.

The first stage of self-tolerance takes place in the thymus (for T cells) and in the bone marrow (for B cells); this is called **central tolerance**. The second stage, **peripheral tolerance**, takes place in secondary lymphoid tissues such as the spleen, lymph nodes, and mucosal lymphoid tissues. Think of central tolerance as a process where autoreactive cells (cells that attack self) are eliminated; and peripheral tolerance as an immunological response that deals with the autoreactive cells that escaped central tolerance.

CENTRAL TOLERANCE – T CELLS

During the maturation of T cells in the thymus, certain T cells become capable of reacting to "self-antigen," namely our own proteins/peptides. Such cells are called **autoreactive**

T cells. Central tolerance, by a process known as **negative selection**, eliminates (kills) such cells before they are released from the thymus (**Fig. 5-1**). Negative selection is useful, since it destroys most high affinity autoreactive T cells.

A subset of autoreactive T cells, with less affinity for self-antigen, changes to cells known as **T regulatory cells** (**T$_{reg}$ cells**), which migrate to the peripheral tissues where they help to maintain peripheral tolerance (described below).

Positive selection, on the other hand, is a process that ensures that mature T cells recognize non-self peptide/ MHC complex.

PERIPHERAL TOLERANCE – T CELLS

This type of self-tolerance is responsible for maintenance of tolerance in secondary lymphoid tissues. Peripheral tolerance works in several ways: **deletion (apoptosis)**, **anergy**, and **suppression**.

- **Deletion** is a process of deleting (killing) the autoreactive cells. It is also called **apoptosis**.
- **Anergy** is the state in which T cells become unresponsive to the antigen stimulation, due to inadequate activation of T cells.
- **Suppression. T regulatory cells**, found in thymus and peripheral tissues, inhibit (suppress) the functions and activation of effector T cells. Such immune response inhibition makes the autoreactive T cells unable to attack self-antigens.

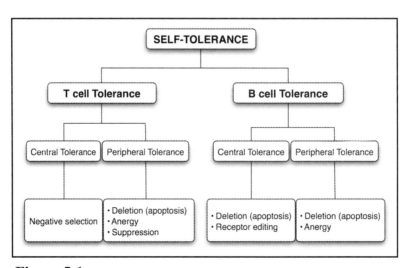

Figure 5-1

CENTRAL AND PERIPHERAL TOLERANCE – B CELLS

During the maturation of B cells in bone marrow, B cells, like T cells in the thymus, may grow to recognize self-antigens. These cells are known as **autoreactive B cells**. As is the case for T cells, there are two parts to self-tolerance for B cells: central and peripheral tolerance.

In **central B tolerance**, autoreactive cells may be deleted (apoptosis) as discussed earlier. They may also change their specificity toward self-antigens. This process is called **receptor editing**, which involves reactivation of certain genes, resulting in expression of a new Ig light chain; this gives the autoreactive cells new specificity. Such changes make the autoreactive cells non-reactive toward self-antigens.

In **peripheral B cell tolerance**, when the autoreactive B cells encounter self-antigen, they are stimulated, but in the absence of T helper cells they become either unresponsive to self-antigen (anergic) or die (apoptosis). Therefore the role of T cell tolerance in maintaining peripheral B cell tolerance is crucial.

FACTORS PREDISPOSING TO AUTOIMMUNITY

Autoimmunity is a result of failure of self-tolerance. When, for any reason, self-tolerance is compromised, autoreactive lymphocytes react to self-antigens and cause tissue damage (autoimmunity) and, eventually, autoimmune diseases.

Genetics and environment are two predisposing factors to autoimmune disease. The **genetic factor** includes HLA (human leukocyte antigen) class I and II genes. HLAs are the genetic designation for the Major Histocompatibility Complex (MHC)(see Chapter 3). The study of HLA genes has revealed that certain autoimmune diseases affect individuals of specific HLA allotypes. For example, there is a greater chance for individuals who carry DR3 and DR4 to develop insulin-dependent diabetes mellitus than individuals who lack these HLA alleles. Also, individuals who carry B27 HLA allele have a greater chance of developing ankylosing spondylitis than those who lack the allele.

An example of a non-MHC gene involved in autoimmunity is the **Fas** gene. The defect in the Fas gene (caused by mutation) impairs the apoptosis of autoreactive B and T cells. This is associated with a human autoimmunity disease known as **Autoimmune Lymphoproliferative Syndrome (ALPS)**.

Environmental predisposing factors include infection, such as *group A Streptococci* and rheumatic fever (discussed later in this chapter). Therefore MHC genes, non-MHC genes, and environmental factors are involved in the production of autoreactive T and B cells. Autoreactive CD4+ T cells that can cause cell-mediated organ damage directly or in conjunction with CD8+ T cells play the central role in autoimmune reactions. Autoreactive B cells, with the help of autoreactive CD4+ T cells, produce IgG autoantibody and cause autoantibody organ damage (**Fig. 5-2**).

MECHANISMS OF AUTOIMMUNITY

Various mechanisms explain how the breakdown of our self-tolerance leads to autoimmune diseases:

1. **Molecular mimicry.** Certain bacteria have two types of **antigenic determinants** (the area of an antigen that is recognized by an antigen receptor). One resembles the structure of self-antigen and the other resembles non self-antigen. Our immune system reacts to both determinants. In other words, our T helper cells help the B cells produce specific antibody against the non self-antigen (the bacterial antigen) and autoantibody against self-antigen, leading to autoimmune disease (**Fig. 5-3**).

   T cells help the B cells to produce both types of antibodies. The best example of molecular mimicry is rheumatic fever. This disease is caused by *Streptococcus pyogenes*, a group A beta hemolytic streptococcus. These bacteria have antigenic determinants that mimic the structure of several host tissues,

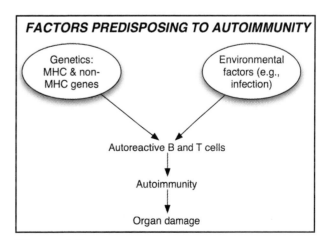

Figure 5-2

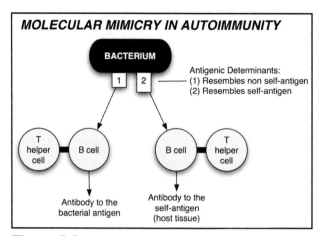

Figure 5-3

including heart, heart valves, and nerve cell membranes. While B cells produce antibody against the streptococcal infection, they also produce antibody against heart tissues, valves and nerve cells. Such attacks target cardiac myosin, tropomyosin, laminin, vimentin, keratin, and N-acetylglucosamine. Valvular involvement includes the mitral valve (common), aortic valve, and the tricuspid valve (uncommon). The natural history of rheumatic fever may include pancarditis (inflammation of epicardium, myocardium, and endocardium), heart failure, and death.

2. **Polyclonal lymphocyte activation. Polyclonal activators** are molecules that can activate B and T cells. Common polyclonal activators of T cells include plant proteins known as **lectins**, such as concanavalin-A and phytohemaglutinin (PHA). Examples of B cell polyclonal activators include anti-Ig antibodies, cytomegalovirus (CMV), and Epstein-Barr viruses. Polyclonal activators activate B and T cells, and since they are not specific, there is a chance of activating autoreactive cells, leading to autoimmune reactions.

3. **Injury and release of sequestered antigens.** Injury to certain tissues, such as the brain, may release antigens into the blood circulation that otherwise would not be recognized.

4. **Antigen spreading.** Autoreactive T and B cells initially recognize a single self-antigen. During progression of the disease, possibly as a result of an inflammatory process, other T and B cells are recruited that would recognize and react to other self-antigens (spreading). As a result of antigen spreading, multiple self-antigens become targets of autoreactivity.

AUTOIMMUNE DISEASES

Autoimmune diseases are the end results of failed self-tolerance. Such diseases are either organ-specific or systemic. A good example of an organ-specific autoimmune disease is Hashimoto thyroiditis. Examples of systemic diseases are Systemic Lupus Erythematosus (SLE), rheumatoid arthritis (RA), systemic sclerosis, and Sjogren syndrome (discussed later in this chapter). **Fig. 5-4** lists examples of autoimmune diseases and associated autoantibodies.

Autoimmunity is the underlying cause of some major rheumatic diseases (**Fig. 5-5**). Note that a person with one rheumatic disease may be at risk for other rheumatic diseases.

Diagnosis of Autoimmune Diseases

Diagnosis of autoimmune diseases is mainly based on clinical grounds. The laboratory workup, including detection of serum autoantibodies, and imaging studies, such as X-rays, help to confirm the diagnosis. It is important to correlate the clinical presentation of the patient with the laboratory findings and imaging studies. One of the hallmarks of laboratory diagnosis is the presence of autoantibodies; some of these autoantibodies are common to a number of autoimmune diseases. However, some may be more specific to one disease than another. For example, antinuclear antibody

---

FIGURE 5-4

Examples of Autoimmune Disease and Associated Autoantibodies

Disease (organ specific)	Organ	Antigen (autoantibody)
Hashimoto throiditis	Thyroid gland	Thyroglobulin, thyroid pcroxidase
Graves disease	Thyroid gland	Thyroid stimulating hormone receptor
Diabetes Type 1	Pancreas	Beta cell antigens
Goodpasture syndrome	Kidney/lungs	Type IV collagen
Pernicious anemia	Gastrointestinal tract	Intrinsic factor, parietal cells
Myasthenia gravis	Muscle	Acetylcholine receptor
Multiple sclerosis	Brain, spinal cord	Myelin proteins
Rheumatic fever	Heart	Myocardial antigens (The antigen is streptococcal group A antigen. However, autoantibody cross reacts with cardiac muscle.)
Addison disease	Adrenal gland	Cytoplasmic P450 antigens
Autoimmune hepatitis	Liver	Hepatocyte antigens

Disease (non-organ specific)	Organ	Antigen
Systemic Lupus Erythematosus (SLE)	Multiple organs	Nuclear and ribosomal antigens
Rheumatoid arthritis	Multiple organs	IgG and nuclear antigens
Systemic sclerosis	Multiple organs	Nucleolar antigens
Polymyositis Dermatomyositis	Multiple organs	Nuclear antigens
Sjogren syndrome	Multiple organs	Cytoplasmic and nuclear antigens

---

(ANA) is detected in the majority of patients with SLE and rheumatoid arthritis, but may also be found in other autoimmune diseases. This antibody attacks a specific component of the cell nucleus. Detection of this antibody using fluorescent staining, a tagged fluorescent antibody against antibody, creates a pattern that gives us a clue as to the type of immune disorder. Therefore, it is important to know the pattern of detected ANA.

The four patterns of ANA include **peripheral (rim)**, **nucleolar**, **speckled**, and **homogeneous**. Some ANA patterns are disease-specific, while others may be common in several diseases. For example, ANA with the speckled pattern is usually seen in patients with Sjogren syndrome, while the ANA with the nucleolar pattern to nucleolus-specific RNA is commonly seen in patients with scleroderma. Another important piece of information is the titer of the ANA.

The titer shows the amount of autoantibody. A high titer, correlated with the clinical picture, may reflect the severity of the disease. **Figure 5-6** summarizes the ANA patterns, the target antigens, and the associated diseases.

Note that the presence of autoantibody does not necessarily mean the presence of autoimmune disease. Autoantibody is usually required but is not sufficient for the diagnosis.

The following are brief discussions of Hashimoto thyroiditis (an example of organ specific disease) and SLE, RA, systemic sclerosis, and Sjogren syndrome (examples of systemic autoimmune diseases).

Hashimoto Thyroiditis
Hashimoto thyroiditis is a chronic autoimmune disease of the thyroid gland. It predominates in women, with a

FIGURE 5-5

Examples of Rheumatic Diseases with Autommune Pathogenesis

Rheumatic disease	Association with other rheumatic diseases
Systemic lupus erythematosus (SLE)	Hemolytic anemia, thyroiditis, idiopathic thrombocytopenic purpura
Rheumatoid arthritis (RA)	SLE, systemic sclerosis (scleroderma)
Polymyositis Dermatomyositis	Sjogren syndrome, SLE, systemic sclerosis
Sjogren syndrome (secondary)	RA, SLE, systemic sclerosis (scleroderma)
Relapsing panniculitis (Weber-Christian disease)	RA, SLE, diabetes mellitus
Relapsing polychondritis	RA, SLE, Sjogren Syndrome

female to male ratio of 10:1. The pathological hallmark of the disease is replacement of the thyroid tissue with lymphocytes, mainly B cells and CD4+ T cells. In the early stage of the disease, patients have a normal level of thyroid hormone (euthyroid). As the disease progresses, the patient develops hyperthyroidism (increased level of serum thyroid hormone) due to release of thyroid hormones by the thyroid tissue. Eventually, patients develop hypothyroidism (low level of thyroid hormone). As the disease progresses, there is gradual destruction of the thyroid tissue by antithyroid antibodies (antithyroglobulin antibody and antimicrosomal antibody).

Diagnosis is based on clinical presentation and laboratory findings. The disease causes various abnormalities (**Fig. 5-7**).

In addition to the detection of autoantibodies, thyroxin hormone (T4) and Thyroid Stimulating Hormone (TSH) may be normal (in the subclinical stage) or abnormal (high TSH and low T4) in the chronic stage of the disease.

Treatment of Hashimoto thyroiditis consists of hormone replacement for hypothyroidism and medication to suppress goiter, if present.

FIGURE 5-6

Antinuclear Antibodies: Patterns and Disease Association

Fluorescein pattern	Target antigens and associated diseases
Peripheral (rim) pattern	Double-stranded DNA (SLE, drug-induced lupus)
Nucleolar pattern	• Nucleolus-specific RNA (sclerodema) • PM-Scl (polymysositis)
Speckled pattern	• Centromere (scleroderma, CREST syndrome, primary biliary cirrhosis) • Jo-1 (polydermatomyositis) • Mi-2 (dermatomyositis) • RANA (rheumatoid arthritis) • RNP (SLE, Sjogren syndrome, scleroderma, rheumatoid arthritis, polymyositis) • Scl-70 (scleroderma) • Sm (SLE) • SS-A (Sjogren syndrome, SLE, heart block, other systemic diseases) • SS-B (Sjogren syndrome, SLE, chronic active hepatitis)
Homogeneous pattern	DNA-histone complexes (SLE, drug-induced lupus, rheumatoid arthritis)

SLE: Systemic Lupus Erythematosus
Sm: Smith antigen
RNP: Ribonucleoprotein
SS-A: also known as Ro
SS-B: also known as La
RANA: Rheumatoid-Associated Nuclear Antigen

FIGURE 5-7

Signs and Symptoms of Hashimoto Thyroiditis

Affected areas	Abnormalities
Weight	Weight again
Thyroid gland	Enlargement (goiter)
Skin	Dry, pale, yellowish color of skin (not common); peripheral and periorbital edema
Nails	Brittle
Hair	Coarse, brittle, thin; hair loss
Cardiovascular	Bradycardia, reduced myocardial contractility, reduced cardiac output, increased diastolic blood pressure, pericardial effusion
Lungs	Respiratory muscle weakness, pleural effusion
Nervous system	Delayed reflexes
Psychiatric	Depression
Gastrointestinal	Constipation
Metabolism	Decreased
Musculoskeletal	Myalgia, arthralgia
Reproductive system	Irregular menstruation
General effect	Fatigue, lethargy, weakness

SLE is a systemic disease that may involve several organs (**Fig. 5-8**). The prognosis depends on the extent of organ involvement.

Treatment of SLE depends on the severity of the disease and the organs involved. Treatment ranges from nonsteroid anti-inflammatory drugs (NSAIDs) to systemic corticosteroids and immunosuppressive medications.

Rheumatoid Arthritis
Rheumatoid arthritis is a chronic inflammatory autoimmune disease of unknown etiology that affects joints and synovial membranes. Infectious agents have been suspected of initiating the synovial inflammation. The theory of bacterial or viral infection etiology, however, has never been proved. A predisposing factor is likely in certain individuals. The disease is associated with several major histocompatibility alleles, mainly DR4. In fact, the majority of patients with RA have a HLA-DR4 haplotype. The immunological hallmark of the disease is production of autoantibodies to IgG, IgM, and IgA, known as **rheumatoid factors** (**RF**). These antibodies recognize and bind to the Fc portion of IgG. RFs are not exclusive to rheumatoid arthritis; they may be found in other diseases, such as mixed cryoglobulinemia, subacute bacterial endocarditis, Lyme disease, and many others. RFs are also found in normal individuals. Rheumatoid factors that bind to IgG form immune complexes that activate the complement system, causing destruction of cell membranes. RA also destroys cartilage after lymphocytes enter the synovial fluid. Lymphocytes produce various cytokines and enzymes, such as proteinases and collagenases that destroy cartilage.

Rheumatoid arthritis involves articular and extra-articular areas. Severity of the disease varies among individuals. While in some patients the disease takes a milder course, in others, the disease is progressive and debilitating. **Fig. 5-9** summarizes the involvement of various organs in RA.

The diagnosis of RA is based on clinical findings, laboratory data, and imaging studies. Four of the 7 criteria below confirm the diagnosis:

1. Arthritis of 3 or more joint areas
2. Arthritis of hand joints
3. Symmetrical arthritis
4. Morning stiffness
5. Rheumatoid nodules (subcutaneous nodules on extensor surfaces, bony prominences, or in juxta-articular regions)
6. Presence of rheumatoid factor

Systemic Lupus Erythematosus (SLE)
Systemic Lupus Erythematosus is a chronic inflammatory autoimmune disease of unknown etiology. Although it mostly affects women of childbearing age with a female to male ratio of 5:1, other age groups are also affected. One characteristic of the disease is the production of autoantibodies to various components of cells. These autoantibodies include antinuclear antibody (ANA), present in over 95% of affected individuals, and two other antibodies that are exclusive to SLE, one to double-stranded DNA and the other to an RNA-protein complex.

The pathogenesis of SLE involves the formation of immune complexes and their deposition in various tissues, such as the kidney. The deposition of immune complexes in kidney glomeruli causes thickening of basement membranes and, in advanced disease, may cause glomerular sclerosis.

FIGURE 5-8

Affected Organs and Abnormalities in Systemic Lupus Erythematosus

Affected areas	Abnormalities	Note
Skin	• **Malar rash** • Generalized erythema • **Discoid lesions** (discoid lupus) • **Oral ulcer** • Vaginal ulcers • **Photosensitivity**	This is a classic butterfly rash over the malar eminence, tending to spare the nasolabial folds
Renal	**Proteinuria or Cellular casts**	• Persistent proteinuria greater than 0.5 gram per day or greater than 3+ • Majority of patients have kidney involvement
Heart	Myocarditis, endocarditis	
Hematopoetic system	**Hemolytic anemia with reticulocytosis, leukopenia, lymphopenia, or thrombocytopenia**	• Leukopenia (less than 4000/mm³ total or on 2 or more occasions) • Lymphopenia (less than 1500/mm³ on 2 or more occasions) • Thrombocytopenia (less than 100,000/mm³ on 2 or more occasions)
Serosa	**Pleuritis or pericarditis**	
Gastrointestinal system	Vasculitis	
Vascular system	Small vessel vasculitis	
Nervous system	Seizures or psychosis	
Immune system	• **Positive LE cell preparations** or • **Antibody to native DNA in abnormal titer** or • **Anti-Sm antibody** • **Abnormal titer of ANA**	
Musculoskeletal system	**Nonerosive arthritis**	Involvement of 2 or more peripheral joints

Note: The words in bold are criteria for diagnosis of SLE by the American College of Rheumatology (diagnosis of SLE requires 4 of 11 criteria). Sm antigen: an RNA-protein complex

---

7. Imaging studies (showing deformities such as erosion or decalcification). The articular and non-articular involvements are summarized in **Fig. 5-9**.

Treatment of RA includes nonsteroidal anti-inflammatory drugs (NSAIDs), corticosteroids, and disease-modifying anti-rheumatic drugs (DMARDs).

Sjogren Syndrome
Sjogren syndrome is a chronic inflammatory autoimmune disease of the exocrine glands, of unknown etiology. The clinical presentation includes dry eyes (**keratoconjunctivitis sicca**) and dry mouth (**xerostomia**). There are two forms of Sjogren syndrome: **primary** and **secondary**. The difference is that the secondary form is also associated with other

FIGURE 5-9

Involved Articular and Non-Articular Areas in Rheumatoid Arthritis

Affected articular areas	Abnormalities	Note
Joints in general	Morning stiffness in and around the joints	It takes about an hour before complete improvement.
Hands	Inflammation of MCP, PIP	DIP are spared.
Elbows	Inflammation of elbow joints	At times, a subcutaneous nodule may be noted on the extensor surface of the forearm adjacent to the elbow.
Shoulder	Decreased range of motion	
Knees	Thickening and effusion of synovial membranes	Baker's (popliteal) cyst is a herniation of the knee joint capsule into the popliteal area. Baker's cyst may also develop from collection of fluid in the popliteal area.
Hip	Symptoms (late stages): • Difficulty putting on shoes • Pain in groin • Pain in buttock • Low back pain	No symptoms at early stages

Affected extra-articular areas

Eyes	• Scleritis • Keratoconjunctivitis sicca	Keratoconjunctivitis is secondary to Sjogren syndrome.
Heart	Pericardial effusion	Found in 50% of patients
Lungs	• Inflammation of cricoarytenoid joint • Pleural effusion • Rheumatic nodule • Diffuse interstitial fibrosis	Laryngeal pain, dysphonia and occasional pain during swallowing
Blood	• Hypochromic microcytic anemia • Felty syndrome	• Common • Felty syndrome is a triad of rheumatoid arthritis, splenomegaly and neutropenia.
Nervous system	• Carpal tunnel • Tarsal tunnel	• Due to entrapment of median nerve at wrist • Due to entrapment of anterior tibial nerve at ankle

MCP = metacarpophalangeal
DIP = Distal Interphalangeal
PIP = Proximal Interphalangeal

autoimmune diseases, such as SLE, RA, and systemic sclerosis. Factors such as elevated rheumatoid factor (>1:320), elevated antinuclear antibody (>1:32), or the presence of anti SS-A (RO) or anti-SS-B (La) antibodies reflect the autoimmune nature of Sjogren syndrome.

Systemic Sclerosis (Scleroderma)

Scleroderma is a chronic disease of unknown etiology that may affect either the skin alone (**localized scleroderma**) or internal organs as well (**systemic sclerosis**). The presence of ANA (topoisomerase I, formerly Scl-70) and RF demonstrate the immunologic nature of the disease. The clinical presentation of the disease includes symmetrical inflammation of the hands and fingers with tightening and hardening of the skin. The skin condition may include other parts of the body, such as the face (mask-like appearance), neck, and trunk. The disease may also involve internal organs such as the lungs, resulting in bibasilar pulmonary fibrosis. Other involved areas may include the heart (**cor pulmonale** and **myocardial fibrosis**) and gastrointestinal system (dysphagia, gastroesophageal reflux, bloating, and diarrhea or constipation).

CHAPTER 6.   COMMON DIAGNOSTIC TESTS

Immunodiagnostic tests are those that detect antigens, antibodies, or antigen-antibody complexes in the body's cells, tissues, and sera, or on the surface membranes of organisms. There are several ways to categorize these tests. The simplest classification divides the tests into **in vitro** tests (tests performed in the laboratory) and **in vivo** tests (tests performed in the host).

IN VIVO TESTING

The common in vivo tests include **prick skin tests, intradermal tests, food challenge tests, protein purified derivative (PPD)** test, and the **patch test (Fig. 6-1)**.

Clinical applications of prick skin testing include allergic rhinitis (see Chapter 4), food allergy (a Type I hypersensitivity to specific food; see Chapter 4), and insect allergies (a Type I hypersensitivity that develops in susceptible individuals when exposed to insect allergens).

Prick Skin Testing

Prick skin testing detects specific IgE antibodies to pollen, mold, pet, food, and insect allergens. Exposure of the allergen to the host causes B cells to differentiate and produce specific IgE to the offending allergen. Later, the specific IgE binds to mast cells. Repeated exposure of the host to the same allergen sensitizes the mast cells and causes the release of mediators, including histamine. Histamine release causes the wheal and flare reaction (a positive test; see Chapter 4). **Fig. 6-2** describes prick skin testing.

Intradermal Testing

Intradermal testing is used for allergic rhinitis and insect allergy (see prick testing above). It is described in **Fig. 6-3**.

Provocative In Vivo Tests

Provocative in vivo tests replicate the natural reaction to an allergen. They have various clinical applications, such as

- an oral food challenge in patients with food allergy
- reproducing asthma, in patients suspicious of asthma
- allergic skin conditions such as **urticaria** (red, raised pruritic skin reaction) and **angioedema** (angio: blood vessel; edema: swelling).

Provocative in vivo tests provoke the host to release histamine. A positive reaction is an immune response identical to the natural host exposure to the offending agent.

FIGURE 6-1

Examples of In Vivo Testing

In vivo test	Mechanism	Clinical applications
Prick skin testing	IgE mediated (Type I hypersensitivity)	Allergic rhinitis, food allergy
Intradermal testing	IgE mediated (Type I hypersensitivity)	Allergic rhinitis
Oral food challenge	IgE mediated (Type I hypersensitivity)	Food allergy
PPD testing	Cell-mediated (Type IV hypersensitivity)	Tuberculosis
Patch testing	Cell-mediated (Type IV hypersensitivity)	Allergic contact dermatitis

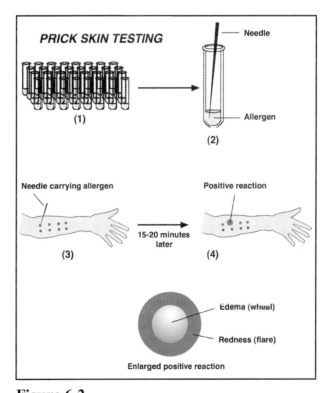

Figure 6-2

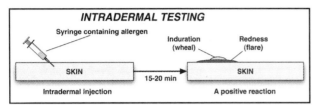

Figure 6-3

FIGURE 6-4

Types of Oral Food Challenge

Type of challenge	Blind
Open label	Neither patient nor physician is blind.
Single blind	Patient is blind.
Double blind placebo controlled	Patient and physician are blind.

In an **open label** challenge (**Fig. 6-4**), the patient and the physician are both aware of the tested allergen. In a **single blind** challenge, the patient is unaware of the nature of the tested allergen (does not know what food allergen is being tested). In a **double blind placebo controlled** challenge (the gold standard), neither the physician nor the patient is aware of the tested food allergen (the food sample is prepared by the physician assistant). The patient is fed (challenged) with each food sample (the suspected food and the placebo, one at a time); then, after each ingestion the reaction is recorded. After completion of the food challenge, the physician breaks the labels and matches the patient's reaction (if any) to the tested food.

Patch Tests

Patch tests are used to test for allergic contact dermatitis from cosmetics, jewelry, pharmaceutical products, cleaning products, and others.

The mechanism of patch testing is a cell-mediated Type IV hypersensitivity (Chapter 4). Patch testing is described in **Fig. 6-5**.

IN VITRO TESTING

In vitro testing is a laboratory technique used to detect a specific antigen, antibody, or antigen-antibody complex in the patient's blood sample (serum or plasma) or tissues.

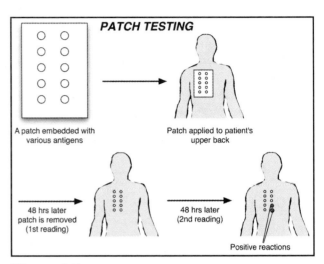

Figure 6-5

Some of the common in vitro tests and their clinical applications, mechanisms, and descriptions are listed in **Fig. 6-6**.

Enzyme-Linked Immunosorbent Assay (ELISA)

ELISA is a test that detects antigen or antibody by using a secondary enzyme-linked antibody. Addition of a chromogenic substrate produces color as an identifying marker for the binding of enzyme-linked second antibody to antigen-antibody complex. There are several variations of ELISA. For example, indirect ELISA, used for detection of HIV, can detect antibody in patient's serum. Sandwich ELISA is another variation of ELISA that detects an unknown antigen (**Fig. 6-7**).

Clinical applications include detection of antibodies in various diseases, such as Human Immunodeficiency Virus (HIV) infection, allergic bronchopulmonary aspergilliosis (ABAP), and autoimmune diseases.

Radioallergosorbent Test (RAST)

RAST is an IgE mediated (Type I hypersensitivity) reaction. The mechanism involves detection of specific IgE antibody in patient's serum with a radiolabeled-conjugated anti IgE antibody (or alternatively, by an enzyme-linked anti IgE antibody) (**Fig. 6-8**).

Clinical applications of RAST, a variation of ELISA, include allergic rhinitis and food allergy.

Western Blotting

The common clinical application of Western blotting is confirmation of an ambiguous HIV test or a positive test by ELISA. **Western blotting** detects anti-HIV antibodies by using gel electrophoresis (a device that separates protein

---

FIGURE 6-6

Examples of In Vitro Testing

Test	Clinical applications
Radioallergosorbent Test (RAST)	Allergic rhinitis, food allergy, insect allergy
Enzyme-Linked Immunosorbent Assay (ELISA)	Detection of HIV antibody
Western blotting	Confirms ambiguous and all positive ELISA tests for HIV
Precipitation	Detects an unknown antigen or an antibody in cells or tissues or on an organism
Agglutination	Detects ABO blood types, Rh antibody, and *Mycoplasma pneumonia* antibody
Immunofluorescence	Detects an unknown antigen, antibody

---

mixtures in an electric field based on their molecular weights and the electric charges) and a second labeled antibody against the patient's serum antibody (**Fig. 6-9**). The advantage of Western blotting as compared to ELISA is that Western blotting is more accurate in matching specific HIV antibodies to specific HIV antigens.

The test ingredients for Western blotting include known HIV antigen(s), the patient's serum, Sodium Dodecyl Sulfate Polyacrylamide Gel (SDS-PAGE) and anti-IgG antibody.

Precipitation

The idea of the **precipitation reaction** is to detect an unknown antigen or antibody by forming a precipitating

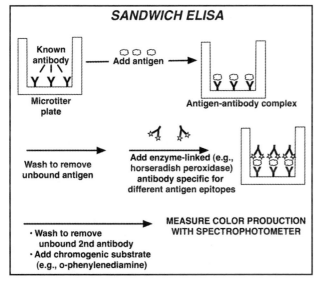

Figure 6-7

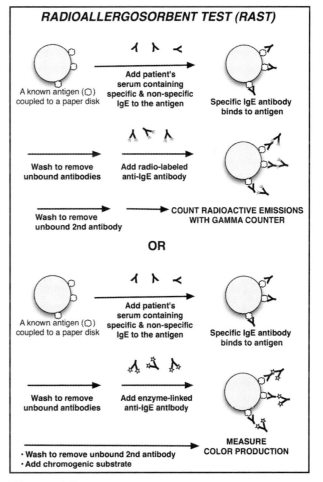

Figure 6-8

antigen-antibody complex. The participating antigens have to have at least 2 antigenic determinants. That is, each antigen should be capable of binding 2 antibodies. Each antibody has 2 binding sites and as a result each antibody can bind 2 antigens. When multiple antigens and antibodies bind to each other, they form a lattice. The lattice is insoluble and precipitates (**Fig. 6-10**).

The precipitation test includes an antigen, an antibody, and serial tubes for mixing antigen and antibody, as follows:

1. Add a fixed amount of antibody to a series of tubes.
2. Add increasing amounts of antigen, starting with tube #1.
3. Observe the precipitate. The maximum binding occurs in the **zone of equivalence** (**Fig. 6-10**).

One example of a precipitation reaction is the **double diffusion** reaction. This reaction can be done in a capillary tube (**Fig. 6-11**) or on a solid phase gel plate (**Ouchterlony reaction**, **Fig. 6-12**). When done in a **capillary tube**, in order to detect an unknown antigen, a fixed amount of an antibody is added to a capillary tube. The antigen and

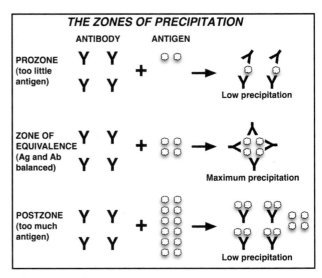

Figure 6-10

antibody diffuse toward each other and form a precipitate, shown as an interphase line in the tube. In the zone of equivalence, a maximum interphase band appears.

In the **Ouchterlony reaction**, one places the antibody in one well and the antigens in two wells opposite the antibody (**Fig. 6-12**). The antigens and antibodies diffuse into the gel, and if the antigens are identical, they form a smooth curve (**line of identity**) between the antigen wells and the antibody well. If different antigens are placed in the wells, then each antigen reacts with the antibody, resulting in lines that cross one another (**lines of non-identity**). If the 2 antigens are similar but not identical, the lines form a spur-like pattern (**lines of partial identity**). The lines formed between antigens and antibodies represent precipitation, and the pattern of lines indicate similarities and dissimilarities of antigens and antibodies.

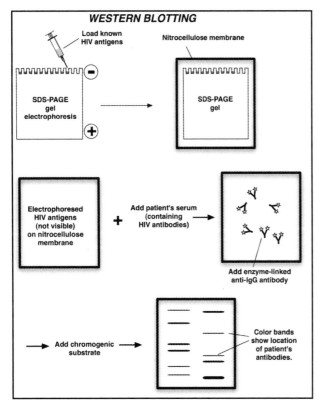

Figure 6-9

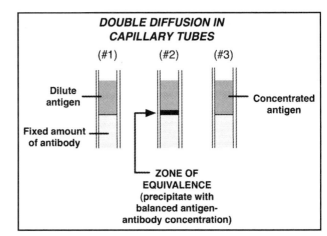

Figure 6-11

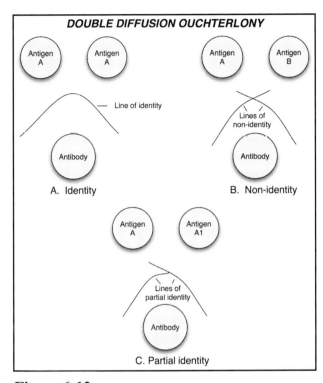

Figure 6-12

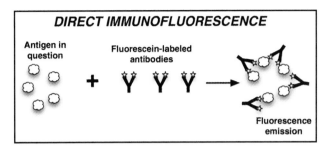

Figure 6-14

Agglutination

The binding of antibody molecules to a particulate antigen (insoluble antigen) causes clumping of the antigen, known as **agglutination**. When antibodies bind to antigens on the surface of red blood cells, the clumping is known as **hemagglutination** (**Fig. 6-13**). The antigen and antibody are referred to as **agglutinogen** and **agglutinin** respectively. The agglutination resulting from direct binding of an antigen and an antibody is known as **direct agglutination**. Agglutination resulting from binding of an antibody to a cell-coated soluble antigen (e.g., red blood cell coated with soluble viral antigen) is known as **indirect agglutination** (**passive agglutination**).

Direct and Indirect Immunofluorescence

In **direct immunofluorescence** reactions, a fluorescent-labeled antibody detects the antigen within a tissue or a cell. The antigen-labeled antibody complex is identified by a fluorescence microscope. The fluorescent dye absorbs light (excitation) and emits detectable light with a certain wavelength (**Fig. 6-14**).

   Indirect immunofluorescence is described in **Fig. 6-15**.

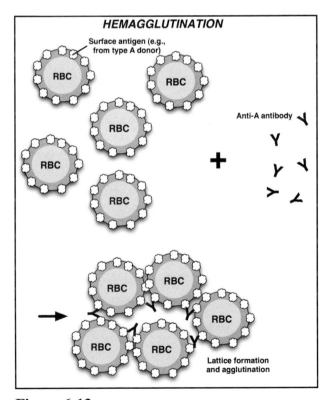

Figure 6-13

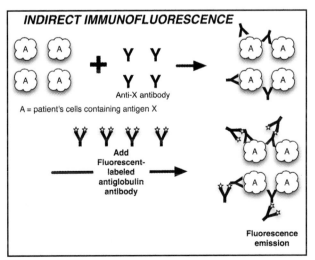

Figure 6-15

CHAPTER 7.   IMMUNODEFICIENCY

Failure of the immune system to perform its normal function results in either **autoimmunity** (Chapter 5) or **immunodeficiency**. **Immunodeficiency** results from decreased function or absence of one or more components of the immune system, which may be **congenital (primary)** or **acquired (secondary)**.

    Primary immunodeficiencies are rare disorders of the immune system in children. They are due to genetic abnormalities (e.g., mutations) that affect various stages of lymphocyte maturation (B or T cells, or both), involving either adaptive immunity or innate immunity (e.g., complement system and phagocytes).

    Acquired immunodeficiencies are relatively common in adults, although they may be seen in children, too. They have various causes, such as immunosuppressive drugs (e.g., cyclosporins used in organ recipients), malnutrition, cancer (bone marrow involvement), radiation therapy (cancer patients), and infections, e.g., Human Immunodeficiency Virus, HIV, in Acquired Immunodeficiency Syndrome (AIDS) (**Fig. 7-1**).

PRIMARY IMMUNODEFICIENCY

Primary immunodeficiencies of the innate immune system include deficiencies affecting the complement system and phagocytes. **Complement deficiencies** are rare but important disorders of the innate immune system; they consist of deficiencies of complement, their receptors, or regulatory factors. Deficiencies of certain components of the complement system are associated with a specific group of diseases and conditions (**Fig. 7-2**).

    Hereditary angioedema is due to deficiency of **C1 esterase inhibitor (C1 INH)**. This regulatory enzyme is an analog of C1r and C1s substrate (C1 has 3 components: C1q, C1r, and C1s). C1q binds to antigen-antibody complex to activate complement; then, the C1r and C1s become activated and bind to C1q. C1 INH binds to C1r and C1s and dissociates them from C1q. Since C1r and C1s are proteolytic components, C1 INH, by this association, regulates the activation of the classic complement system (**Fig. 7-3**).

    Another function of C1 INH is inhibition of factor XII (Hageman factor) and kallikrein (two serine proteases in the blood coagulation pathway). Therefore, deficiency of C1 INH affects the activation of the classic complement pathway and blood coagulation, which leads to accumulation of bradykinin (a vasoactive mediator) and accumulation of tissue fluid (edema). The majority of affected individuals have a family history of angioedema. One unique feature of individuals with hereditary angioedema is the absence of urticaria. In general, within an affected population with either urticaria or angioedema, 50% have combined urticaria and angioedema, 40% have urticaria alone, and 10% have angioedema alone.

    The absence of phagocytes or phagocytic function results in failure of the immune system to clear pathogenic organisms, which leads to repeated infections and

---

FIGURE 7-1

Classification of Immunodeficiencies

Immunodeficiency type	Age of onset	Occurrence	Etiology
Congenital (primary)	Usually childhood	Rare	Genetic abnormalities (e.g., mutation) affecting the immune components of innate and or adaptive immunity (e.g., B cells, T cells, the complement system, phagocytes)
Acquired (secondary)	Usually adulthood	Relatively common	• Infections (Human Immunodeficiency Virus) • Immunosuppressive drugs (e.g., cyclosporin) • Metastatic malignancies to the bone • Radiation therapy in cancer patients • Malnutrition • Idiopathic

FIGURE 7-2

Complement Deficiencies and Their Associated Diseases

Complement deficiency	Associated disease
C1-C4	Rheumatoid disorder (e.g., SLE)
C5-C9	Neisserial infections
C1q, C2, C3, C5, C6, C7, C8, C9, factor I, properdin	Recurrent pyogenic infections
Cl esterase inhibitor (Cl INH)	Hereditary angioedema

FUNCTION OF C1 ESTERASE INHIBITOR (C1 INH)

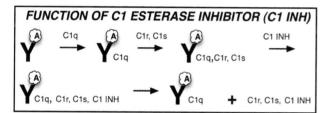

Figure 7-3

sometimes death. In order to combat pathogens, phagocytes need to be in sufficient numbers, migrate to the site of injury, and destroy the invading organisms with lytic enzymes. Deficiency affecting any of the above functions leads to failure of normal phagocytic function. Genetic abnormality affecting myelogenic stem cell precursors can lead to absence of neutrophils (**agranulocytosis**) or reduced neutrophils (**neutropenia**). In **cyclic neutropenia**, the number of neutrophils fluctuates in a 21-day cycle. Acquired causes of neutropenia include chemotherapeutic drugs and radiation in cancer patients (**Fig. 7-4**).

In order for phagoctes and lymphocytes to migrate to the site of injury, they must adhere to the vascular endothelium by one of their surface **adhesion molecules**. Deficiency of such molecules renders the phagocytes unable to attach to the vascular endothelium, with failure to migrate the site of injury (**leukocyte adhesion deficiency syndrome**). Affected individuals may have delayed umbilical cord detachment (due to adhesion defect), poor wound healing, and severe bacterial infections (e.g., pneumonia, otitis media, chronic skin infection).

Phagocytes use their lytic enzymes to destroy engulfed organisms. In **Chronic Granulomatous Disease (CGD)**, there is a defect in phagocyte oxidase (an enzyme that converts oxygen to Reactive Oxygen Intermediates, ROI, e.g., superoxide anion). The result is the lack of ROIs and inability of the phagocyte to destroy the engulfed organisms. Most cases are diagnosed in the first few years of life. Affected individuals are prone to intracellular bacterial and fungal infections, with granulomas (aggregation of phagocytes at the site of injury along with lymphocytes and other cells) in the skin, gastrointestinal, and genitourinary tracts, and with abscesses in the lungs, liver, and spleen.

Immunodeficiency Affecting Adaptive Immunity

Immunodeficiency affecting the adaptive immune system includes an absence or abnormal function of B cells, T cells, or both.

FIGURE 7-4

Immunodeficiency Affecting Phagocytes

Condition	Feature	Outcome
Agranulocytosis	Absence of neutrophils	Absence of this type of cell for participating in phagocytosis
Neutropenia	Reduced neutrophils (<1500)	Inability to fight effectively against organisms due to insufficient number of neutrophils
Leukocyte adhesion deficiency	Defective migration	Inability to move to the injury site due to defective adherence
Chronic granulomatous disease	Defective lytic enzyme	Inability to destroy the engulfed organisms, resulting in susceptibility of affected individuals to bacterial and fungal infection

Immunodeficiency Affecting Humoral Immunity (antibody deficiency)

B cells produce antibodies (immunoglobulins). Therefore, a deficiency of B cells renders the affected individuals prone to infection by encapsulated bacteria (e.g., *Streptococcus pneumonia, Haemophilus influenzae*). This type of immunodeficiency is a result of either an absence of B cells or the inability of B cells to mature, resulting in an absence or low levels of one or more immunoglobulins. Defective T cells may also impede the production of antibodies. Several examples of antibody deficiency are depicted in **Fig. 7-5**.

X-linked agammaglobulinemia
X-linked agammaglobulinemia (Bruton agammaglobulinemia) is the first reported primary immunodeficiency. It results from an inability of B cells to mature; there is a

mutation in enzymes involved in B cell maturation. Affected individuals are devoid of peripheral B cells and have low levels of immunoglobulins. Due to antibody deficiencies, the affected individuals are prone to bacterial sinopulmonary infections (such as *Streptococcus pneumoniae* and *Haemophilus influenzae)* and viral infections with Echo and Coxsackie viruses.

Common variable immunodeficiency
Affected individuals with **common variable immunodeficiency** have normal or decreased B cells but low levels of immunoglobulins. This immunodeficiency disease manifests as early as infancy and as late as late adulthood. Usually IgM, IgG, and IgA are deficient. The function of both B cells and T cells is impaired. Affected individuals are prone to recurrent bacterial infections with *Streptococcus pneumoniae* and *Haemophilus influenzae*.

FIGURE 7-5

Immunodeficiencies Affecting Humoral and Cell-Mediated Immunity

Immunodeficiency	Humoral immunodeficiency (antibody deficiency)	Cell-mediated immunodeficiency (T cell deficiency)	Features	Clinical presentation
X-linked agammaglobulinemia (Bruton's agammaglobulinemia)	+		Absence (or low level) of immunoglobulins	Bacterial infections, viral infections
Common variable immunodeficiency	+		Normal or decreased B cells, reduced immunoglobulins	Bacterial infections, autoimmune diseases
IgA deficiency	+		Absent or reduced IgA	Ranges from asymptomatic to to sinusitis, respiratory infections, and autoimmune diseases
Hyper IgE syndrome (Job syndrome)	+		Significantly high level of IgE, normal level of other Igs	Recurrent infections of skin and lungs (staphylococcal abscess)
DiGeorge syndrome		+	Low T cells, no T cell response	Cardiac and thymic defects, parathyroid dysfunction
Severe Combined Immunodeficiency Disease (SCID)	+	+	Deficiency of B and T cell	Prone to bacterial, viral, and fungal infections
Ataxia telangiectasia, a form of SCID	+	+	As SCID	Ataxia, telangiectasia

IgA deficiency

IgA deficiency is the most common primary immunodeficiency. Affected individuals lack IgA or have a low level of the antibody. The other immunoglobulins may be normal or elevated. Individuals with this immunodeficiency may appear asymptomatic or present with respiratory or gastrointestinal infections. They may have associated IgG2 or IgG4 deficiency.

Hyper Immunoglobulin E (IgE) syndrome

Hyper Immunoglobulin E (IgE) syndrome (Job syndrome) is an autosomal disease of unknown etiology. Affected individuals have a significantly high level of IgE and normal levels of other immunoglobulins. The clinical presentation is recurrent infection of the skin and lungs (Staphyloccal abscess) and eczema.

Immunodeficiency Affecting Cell-mediated Immunity (T cell deficiency)

DiGeorge Syndrome

DiGeorge Syndrome (congenital thymic aplasia) is a prototype of cell-mediated immunodeficiency. The deficiency is due to incomplete development of the thymus from the third and fourth pharyngeal pouches, leading to cardiac and thymic defects and parathyroid dysfunction. Affected individuals have low numbers of T cells and no T cell response, with susceptibility to viral and fungal infections. Patients may have a mild disease with a good prognosis or a severe disease with recurrent infections (**Fig. 7-5**).

Immunodeficiency Affecting Both Humoral and Cell-mediated Immunity (combined B and T cell deficiency)

The prototype for combined B and T cell deficiency is a series of immunodeficiency diseases known as **Severe Combined Immunodeficiency Diseases (SCID)** (**Fig. 7-5**). Affected individuals, being deficient in both B and T cells, are prone to bacterial (e.g., otitis), viral (e.g., Epstein-Barr), and fungal (e.g., candidiasis) infections. If not treated, they die in the first year of life. Examples of SCID include **X-linked SCID**, **autosomal recessive SCID**, and **Adenosine Deaminase** (an enzyme in the purine salvage pathway) **Deficiency (ADA)**.

Ataxia telangiectasia

Ataxia telangiectasia is another example of combined humoral and cell-mediated immunodeficiency. Patients with this multisystem disease present with progressive ataxia (an inability to coordinate muscle activity), leading to problems with walking by age 10-12 years. The other clinical characteristic of this disease is telangiectasia (chronic dilation of capillaries) at 3-6 years of age. These patients are prone to recurrent sinopulmonary infections, autoimmune diseases, and malignancies (e.g., non-Hodgkin lymphoma). The underlying etiology is the mutation of a gene that participates in repair of damaged DNA. The B cell and T cell numbers are normal or reduced. The common immunoglobulin deficiency is IgA, which may be associated with IgG2 and/or IgE deficiency.

SECONDARY (ACQUIRED) IMMUNODEFICIENCY

Secondary (acquired) immunodeficiency is more common than primary immunodeficiency. It results from infections, immunosuppressive medications, malnutrition, and neoplastic diseases. The most common and prevalent secondary immunodeficiency is **Acquired Immunodeficency Syndrome (AIDS)**. The World Health Organization (WHO), in its December 2007 global summary of the AIDS epidemic, reported that in 2007 there were 33.2 million people living with HIV, 2.5 million newly infected with HIV and 2.1 million AIDS deaths. AIDS is a progressive immunodeficiency that leads to various infections by opportunistic organisms (e.g., *Pneumocystis carinii*) and increased malignancies (e.g., lymphoma). AIDS results from infection with **Human Immunodeficiency Virus (HIV)**. HIV is a single-stranded retrovirus RNA (retroviruses are viruses that can make a complementary DNA) that infects the human host cells via exposure to blood or bodily secretions of an infected individual. There are two types of HIV. HIV-1 is the major cause of AIDS. HIV-2 causes a similar syndrome and is prevalent in South Africa and India. The HIV structure consists of a lipid bilayer membrane with 2 glycoprotein projections, gp120 (external) and gp41 (transmembrane), 2 single-stranded RNAs and several enzymes (p32 integrase, p64 reverse transcriptase, and p10 protease) surrounded by a nucleocapsid (p24) and outer membrane (P17) (**Fig. 7-6**).

HIV targets CD4 surface receptors on lymphocytes, but other cells with CD4 receptors, such as macrophages and dendritic cells, are also targets. The basic sequence of events is as follows (**Fig. 7-7**):

1. Gp120 of HIV membranes binds to CD4 receptors of the target cell (e.g., CD4+ T cell). This is known as **fusion**.
2. After penetration of the virus, the RNAs are released into the cytoplasm.

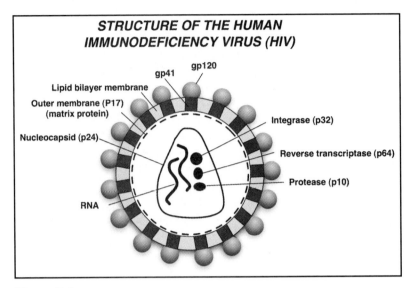

STRUCTURE OF THE HUMAN IMMUNODEFICIENCY VIRUS (HIV)

Figure 7-6

3. With the help of the enzyme **reverse transcriptase**, the RNA makes a complementary copy of DNA (cDNA).
4. The cDNA penetrates the host nucleus and integrates into the host DNA genome with the help of the enzyme **integrase**. At this time the integrated DNA is called **proviral DNA**.
5. The proviral DNA makes messenger RNA (mRNA). This step is known as **transcription**.

6. The mRNA produces viral proteins (**translation**).
7. The single-stranded RNAs, along with the viral protein enzymes, are packaged into membranes and leave the cell. This process is known as **budding** (the nucleus package takes a part of the host membrane and makes an envelope of its own).

The **course of the infection** starts with a **latency period**. In this time, the infected host remains asymptomatic.

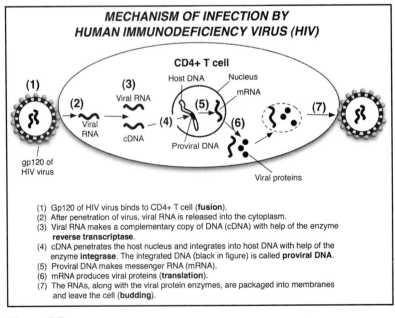

MECHANISM OF INFECTION BY HUMAN IMMUNODEFICIENCY VIRUS (HIV)

(1) Gp120 of HIV virus binds to CD4+ T cell (**fusion**).
(2) After penetration of virus, viral RNA is released into the cytoplasm.
(3) Viral RNA makes a complementary copy of DNA (cDNA) with help of the enzyme **reverse transcriptase**.
(4) cDNA penetrates the host nucleus and integrates into host DNA with help of the enzyme **integrase**. The integrated DNA (black in figure) is called **proviral DNA**.
(5) Proviral DNA makes messenger RNA (mRNA).
(6) mRNA produces viral proteins (**translation**).
(7) The RNAs, along with the viral protein enzymes, are packaged into membranes and leave the cell (**budding**).

Figure 7-7

After a period of months to years, the proviral DNA becomes activated and produces multiple copies of the virus (**propagation**). The viruses leave the cells as described above and infect other cells. Progression of infection leads to destruction of many CD4+ T cells (about 25-60 cells/mm^3 per year), and eventually the patient becomes symptomatic. A variety of hypotheses accounts for the reduction of CD4+ T cells, including apoptosis, direct destruction by HIV, and destruction by cytotoxic CD8+ cells.

The initial symptoms of HIV infections are flu-like symptoms (**viral syndrome**), where patients experience headache, malaise, fever, myalgia, arthralgia, lymphadenopathy, and sore throat. Then, the patients become asymptomatic for months to years. While asymptomatic, the viruses continue propagating and destroying CD4+ T cells. During the latency period, lymphadenopathy persists, and as the infection progresses, more CD4 + T cells are depleted; eventually opportunistic infections complicate the picture. Finally, the progression of the HIV infection leads to AIDS, where the total CD4+ T cell count (normal range 500-1500 cells/mm^3, varying with different laboratories) falls below 200 cells/mm^3 and the affected individual becomes cachectic and infected with opportunistic infections.

DIAGNOSIS OF IMMUNODEFICIENCY

Diagnosis of immunodeficiency starts with obtaining a comprehensive history of the medical illness: the time of onset, the symptoms, the type of infection (bacterial, viral, fungal), and any family history of similar conditions. The initial laboratory workup includes a Complete Blood Count (CBC) and a basic chemistry panel. The CBC may reveal lymphopenia, neutropenia, or thrombocytopenia (**Fig. 7-8**).

The above abnormalities can also result from certain medications (e.g., immunosuppressive drugs used in transplantation). The following is an outline of the workup for immunodeficiencies.

Workup for Primary Immunodeficiencies of the Innate Immune System

Complement deficiencies can be investigated by measuring serum complement levels. Measuring CH50 can indicate complement deficiency, but measuring a specific complement identifies the specific immunodeficiency.

The workup for **immunodeficiency** of **phagocytes** (e.g., neutrophils) consists of measuring serum neutrophil levels. If the neutrophil numbers are normal, then the next step is a neutrophil function assay (an assay to evaluate neutrophil function).

Workup for Primary Immunodeficiencies of the Adaptive Immune System

The workup for **humoral immunity** (**antibody deficiency**) consists of measuring B cells and serum immunoglobulin levels (usually IgA, IgM, IgG and IgE). At times, measuring subclasses of IgG (IgG 1, 2, 3, and 4) is useful, since total IgG sometimes is normal but the affected patient is deficient in an IgG subclass. If the immunoglobulin measurements show reduction, the next step is injecting encapsulated bacteria vaccines such as *Haemophilus influenzae* or the pneumonia vaccine (23 serotypes) and then measuring

---

FIGURE 7-8

Workup of Immunodeficiencies

Immunodeficiency	Workup
All Patients	CBC, chemistry
Deficiencies of innate immunity	Neutrophil count, neutrophil function, complement levels
Antibody deficiency	B cell count, immunoglobulin and IgG subclasses level, antibody function test (injecting pneumonia and influenza vaccines and checking the titer)
Cell-mediated (T cell deficiency)	T cells and subpopulation count, T cell function, cell-mediated skin testing
Secondary immunodeficiencies (HIV infection)	HIV test (ELISA and Western blotting), cell-mediated skin testing

the antibody level in about one month. These levels (23 serotypes) should be compared with pre-vaccine antibody levels to see if there is an increase in the titer. In an **immunocompetent** patient (one with an intact immune system), the 23 serotype antibody titers should increase about 2 to 2 1/2 times the pre-vaccine level. Failure of titer improvements confirms the immunodeficiency.

Workup for primary cell-mediated (T cell deficiency) immunity includes measuring T cells and their subpopulations (specifically CD4+ T cells and CD8+ T cells). An in vivo test consists of skin testing for delayed hypersensitivity. This test is done by injecting an antigen (e.g., *Candida* antigen) intradermally and looking for a delayed reaction. An absence of reaction to *Candida* confirms cell-mediated immunodeficiency.

Workup for the HIV-infected patient includes measuring HIV by ELISA and confirming the positive results with Western blotting (Chapter 6). During the course of infection, total CD4+ T cells and the viral load (the quantitative measurements of viral copies) should be followed.

MANAGEMENT OF IMMUNODEFICIENCY

- Ideally, the immunodeficient patient should **avoid exposure to microorganisms**. The story of the "Bubble Boy" was an example of extreme avoidance. In reality, such circumvention is not practical, but one can try to reduce the exposure level, e.g., wearing a face mask outdoors and in crowded places (**Fig. 7-9**).
- **Genetic counseling** is a logical plan to help manage familial immunodeficiencies.
- **Prophylactic use of antibiotics** as a preventive measure is important in preparing to fight recurrent bacterial infections.
- For certain humoral immunodeficiencies, **Intravenous Immunoglobulin (IVIG)** is an alternative to antibiotics. An IVIG is a pool of gamma globulin from thousands of patients. This pool carries many antibodies, due to its lifelong exposure to various microorganisms.
- In recent years, the introduction of **subcutaneous immunoglobulin** has provided a simpler alternative to IVIG.
- Finally, **bone marrow transplantation** has been reported helpful in several immunodeficiencies, such as Severe Combined Immunodeficiency (SCID) and chronic granulomatous disease.

Management of Acquired Immunodeficiency Syndrome

Management of **Acquired Immunodeficiency Syndrome (AIDS)** requires prophylactic antibiotics for prevention of

---

FIGURE 7-9

Management of Immunodeficiency

Immunodeficiency	Management
All types of immunodeficiencies	Avoidance of microorganisms, or measures to reduce the exposure
Primary immunodeficiencies	Genetic counseling
Antibody deficiencies	Intravenous Immunoglobulin (IVIG)
Severe Combined Immunodeficiency (SCID); chronic granulomatous disease	Bone marrow transplantation
Cell-mediated immunodeficiencies (T cell deficiencies)	Prophylactic antibiotics if necessary
HIV infection/AIDS	Prophylactic antibiotics, HAART
HIV = Human Immunodeficiency Virus	
AIDS = Acquired Immunodeficiency Syndrome	
HAART = Highly Active Anti-Retroviral Therapy	
IVIG = Intravenous immunoglobulin	

opportunistic infections. Controlling viral replication is an important strategy. The following inhibitor drugs work at different sites:

- **Reverse transcriptase inhibitors drugs** are nucleoside analogs that inhibit reverse transcription of the viral RNA to complementary DNA.
- **Protease inhibitor drugs** inhibit cleavage of the proteins necessary for making a new virion.
- **Fusion inhibitors** inhibit attachment of the virus to the target cells.

Therapy is a cocktail of at least 3 medications of different classes (one or two of reverse transcriptase, and one or two of protease inhibitor drugs). This combination is known as **HAART (Highly Active Anti-retroviral Therapy)**. It works by reducing the viral load to a low and undetectable level. Note that HAART is not considered a cure for HIV infection. Research and clinical trials for an HIV/AIDS vaccine are underway nationally and globally. Although some progress has been made, a successful vaccine is still unavailable at the time of this writing.

CHAPTER 8.   VACCINATION

As you recall, in order to eradicate invading microorganisms, we need the innate and the adaptive immune systems. These systems work in concert to confront and remove the foreign invaders. However, the innate system has no memory of previously invading pathogens. The adaptive immune system, though, remembers past exposures (**Fig. 8-1**).

Our immune systems may effectively win the battle with the pathogenic microorganism (e.g., measles virus) or may succumb to a disease (e.g., measles, also known as rubeola). After the natural course of the disease (**natural infection**), the body develops natural immunity against the causative microorganism (e.g., measles virus). There is another way though, that we can protect ourselves. That is an injection of a live **attenuated** (reduced disease-causing capability) microorganism, such as measles virus, into the host which stimulates the adaptive immune system to produce a specific antibody against the virus. Immunity as a result of a natural infection or an inoculation of the causative agent is known as **active immunity**.

The concept of an artificial inoculation of a host with a pathogenic microorganism in order to produce protection is known as **vaccination**, and the inoculated antigen is called **vaccine** (from **vacca**, cow). In 1796, Edward Jenner, an English physician, observed that individuals who contracted cowpox were immune against contracting smallpox. To demonstrate this, he inoculated a young boy with a cowpox pustule and later with the smallpox virus. He noted that the boy did not contract smallpox. This showed that cowpox had caused immunity against small pox. The term **vaccination** was later broadened to include similar protection against other bacteria and viruses.

Another form of immunity, **passive immunity**, refers to a prepared antibody acquired from the mother (via placenta during pregnancy, or from breast-feeding during lactation), pooled donor antibodies, e.g., administration of an Intravenous Gamma Globulin (IVIG), or a specific antibody. One type of active immunization (vaccination) and one type of passive immunization (IVIG) are discussed in the following sections.

IMMUNE RESPONSE TO VACCINATION

The first immune response to the infective microorganism (either natural or artificial inoculation) is known as the **primary immune response**. This starts after a **lag period**, the time period (several days to a week, depending on the pathogen) from inoculation of the microorganism until the appearance of the antibody. The lag period is followed by a surge and then a decrease in the antibody titer. The major antibody in the primary immune response is IgM. When the host is later injected with the same pathogen, the immune response is known as the **secondary immune response**, which has a shorter lag period. This is due to the presence of a significant number of memory cells. The major antibody in the secondary immune response is IgG. The antibody surge reaches a higher peak than the first immune response peak, lasts longer, and has higher affinity for the antigen than in the primary immune response (**Figs. 8-2, 8-3**).

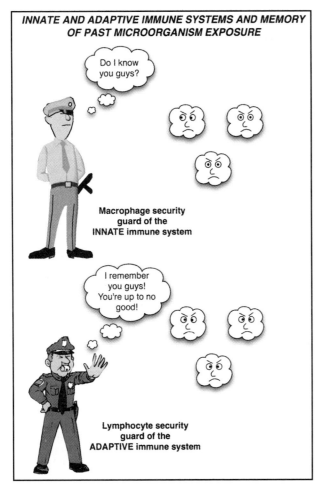

Figure 8-1

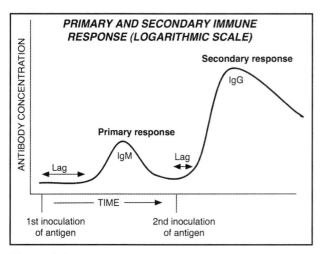

Figure 8-2

TYPES OF VACCINES

Ideally, we should have a vaccine with one method of preparation for every known infectious disease. In reality, though, preparation of vaccine is only possible for a few diseases; this is because the smart microorganisms change their structures (mutation) and frequently appear as new organisms. The following are different types of vaccine preparation.

- **In live attenuated vaccine** preparation, the microorganism's pathogenicity has been attenuated. This form of microorganism (virus or bacterium) cannot cause the disease; immunocompromised patients, however, are exceptions and may contract the disease. The immunity post-vaccination is long-lasting and may be lifelong.
- **Killed-bacteria vaccine** stimulates the immune system to produce protective antibodies, without causing the disease. The protection by this type of preparation is shorter than that of live viral vaccines. Some vaccines (**subunit**

vaccines) are purified macromolecules such as bacterial toxins, bacterial polysaccharides, or bacterial DNA.

- **Toxoid vaccines** are preparations of weakened bacterial exotoxins that, while producing protection in the host, do not cause the disease (e.g., diphtheria and tetanus toxoid vaccines).
- **Bacterial polysaccharide vaccines** are preparations of bacterial polysaccharides (e.g., polysaccharides of *Streptococcus pneumoniae* and *Haemophilus influenzae*). Bacterial polysaccharides cannot stimulate the T helper response on their own; therefore, they are conjugated with a protein carrier. In this way, the **conjugated vaccine** can stimulate T helper cells and activate T cell dependent antibody production. An example is conjugation of bacterial polysaccharide with the toxoid of *Haemophilus influenzae* (**Fig. 8-4**).
- **Allergy immunotherapy** is also a form of **vaccination**. In 1997, the Word Health Organization (WHO) met in Geneva and released a position paper proposing that the term "vaccine" refer to allergen extracts used in allergen immunotherapy. It makes sense because allergens include proteins extracted from pollens, dust mites, pets, molds and insects; they stimulate the production of specific antibodies and in a sense are similar to traditional bacterial and viral vaccinations.

We are constantly exposed to small amounts of pollens, pet danders, and dust mites in our environment. Although our immune system can fight against a small amount of such allergens, our defense system is not prepared to confront large amounts (i.e., high pollen counts) of aeroallergens. The role of allergy immunotherapy is the building up of immunity against specific allergens. Such immunity reduces or eliminates symptoms associated with the exposed allergen.

One would think that administration of an allergy vaccine may worsen the allergy symptoms. Fortunately,

---

FIGURE 8-3

Characteristics of the Primary and Secondary Immune Response

Immune response	Lag phase	Antibody titer	Antibody affinity	Duration of antibody availability	Major antibody
Primary	Longer	Lower	Lower	Shorter	IgM
Secondary	Shorter	Higher	Higher	Longer	IgG

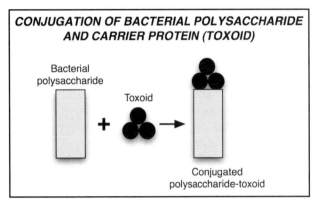

CONJUGATION OF BACTERIAL POLYSACCHARIDE AND CARRIER PROTEIN (TOXOID)

Bacterial polysaccharide

Toxoid

Conjugated polysaccharide-toxoid

Figure 8-4

FIGURE 8-5

Characteristic of an Ideal Vaccine

Characteristic	Comment
Safety	Lack of disease-causing capability, absence or low adverse reactions
Immunity	Protects the recipient
Long-lasting protection	Years to lifelong
High specificity	Protection against a specific disease
Ease of administration	Increased compliance
Cost effectiveness	To individuals and to mass recipients

this is not the case. Injection of vaccine starts with administration of a small amount of allergen (subcutaneous injection). This is followed by weekly increases of the allergen dose. After each injection, the patient is monitored for a possible allergic reaction. After approximately 4-6 months, the vaccine does reaches a **maintenance dose** level. After reaching the maintenance dose, vaccination frequency changes to 2-4 week intervals and the administered dose remains the same until completion of immunotherapy, which may take 3-5 years.

Several immunological changes take place during allergy vaccination. Allergy immunotherapy induces the production of allergen-specific antibody. This IgG antibody, also known as **blocking antibody**, competes with IgE. Other changes during allergy vaccination include shifting of the Th2 CD4+ T cells to Th1 CD4+ T cells and reduction of mediator release from mast cells and basophils. A successful allergy vaccination is associated with immune tolerance, in which the immune system reduces the immune response to a specific allergen. Therefore, allergy vaccination does not worsen the symptoms and, like other vaccines, boosts our immunity to specific allergens.

CHARACTERISTICS OF AN IDEAL VACCINE

An ideal vaccine has the following characteristics (**Fig. 8-5**):

- **Safety.** The vaccine should not cause a disease or an adverse reaction in the recipient.
- **Immunity.** The preparation should stimulate the immune system to produce immunity against a specific disease.
- **Long-lasting protection** (years to lifelong) against a specific disease

- **High specificity**
- **Ease of administration**, which increases compliance
- **Cost effectiveness**

Contraindications to vaccination are listed in **Fig. 8-6**.

RECOMMENDED VACCINES FOR CHILDREN AND ADULTS

The Center for Disease Control (CDC) has recommended the following vaccination schedules for children and adults, shown in **Fig. 8-7**, **Fig. 8-8**, and **Fig. 8-9**.

Two examples of vaccines used in children and adults (pneumococcal vaccine and HPV vaccine) and one example of an adult vaccine (shingles) are summarized below.

Pneumococcal vaccine

Pneumococcal bacteria cause pneumonia, bacteremia, and meningitis. Vaccination is the best way to prevent these devastating diseases. Pneumococcal vaccine is a subunit vaccine pooled from 23 types of pneumococcal bacteria. It is indicated in patients age 2 or older with chronic diseases (e.g., diabetes mellitus, cardiovascular disease, chronic renal failure, nephrotic syndrome). It is also indicated for those with asplenia, residents of nursing homes, certain ethnic groups (perhaps due to alcohol abuse, HIV, sickle cell disease, poverty or environment; e.g., Alaska

FIGURE 8-6

Contraindications to Vaccination

Condition	Example	Comment
Immunocompromised patients	Acquired Immunodeficiency Syndrome (AIDS)	Avoid live vaccine preparations.
Cancer patients	Lymphoma, leukemia	Avoid live vaccine preparations.
Pregnancy	Anytime during gestation	Avoid live vaccine preparations.
Allergy (food)	Allergy to egg, chicken	Avoid chick embryo cell culture vaccines (e.g., measles and mumps vaccines). Avoid embryonated chicken egg vaccines (e.g., influenza).
Allergy	Allergy to any components of the vaccines	Avoid the vaccine containing allergenic ingredients.

FIGURE 8-7

Center for Disease Control (CDC) Recommended Vaccine Schedule for Children Ages 0-6 Years

Vaccine	Age	Total doses
Hepatitis A (Hep A)	12-23 months	2 doses 6 months apart
Hepatitis B (Hep B)	At birth, 1-2 months, and 6-18 months	3
Rotavirus (Rota)	At 2, 4, and 6 months	3
Diphtheria, Tetanus, Pertussis (DTaP)	At 2, 4, 6, 15-18 months, and 4-6 years	5
Haemophilus influenza type b (Hib)	2, 4, 6, and 12-15 months	4
Pneumococcal (pneumococcal conjugate vaccine, PCV)	2, 4, 6, and 12-15 months	4
Pneumoccocal (pneumococcal polysaccharide vaccine, PPV) for certain high risk groups	2-6 years	1
Inactivated poliovirus (IPV)	2, 4, 6-18 months, and 4-6 years	4
Influenza	6-59 months and annually after 5 years of age if have high risk	1 dose; but for children under 9 years who receive it for the first time, 2 doses at least 4 weeks apart
Measles, Mumps, Rubella (MMR)	12-15 months and 4-6 years	2
Varicella	12-15 months and 4-6 years	2
Meningococcal (Meningococcal Conjugate Vaccine, MCV4)	2-6 years	1

FIGURE 8-8

**Center for Disease Control (CDC) Recommended Vaccine Schedule for
Persons Ages 7-18 Years**

Vaccine	Age	Total doses	Note
Hepatitis A (Hep A)	7-18 years	2, six months apart	This vaccine is indicated for certain high-risk groups.[1]
Hepatitis B (Hep B)	7-18 years	3 doses	The series is for those who were not previously vaccinated.
Tetanus and diphtheria toxoids and acellular pertussis (Tdap)	11-12 years	1	Those who did not receive the vaccine may receive it at 13-18 years.
Human Papillomavirus (HPV)	11-12 years	3	Administer the second dose a month after the first dose and the third dose 6 months after the first dose. Those who did not receive it at 11-12 years of age may receive the series at 13-18 years.
Meningococcal (MCV4)	11-12 years	1	Those not previously vaccinated may receive the vaccine at age 13-18 years. Certain high-risk groups may receive the vaccine at age 2-10 years.
Pneumococcal	7-18 years	1	Certain high-risk groups[1]
Influenza	7-18 years	1	Yearly vaccine to certain high-risk groups[1]
Inactivated Poliovirus (IPV)	Over 7 years	1	If the individual received the series and third dose was administered at age 4 or older, then the fourth dose is not needed.
Measles, Mumps, Rubella (MMR)	7-18 years	2	Those who were not previously vaccinated should receive 2 doses at least 4 weeks apart.
Varicella	7-18 years	2	Less than 13 years, 2 doses at least 3 months apart. Over 13 years, 2 doses at least 4 weeks apart

(1) On the basis of medical, occupational, life style, or other indications.

natives, African Americans, certain native Americans), healthcare providers, and individuals 65 years or older. The recommended schedule is 1-2 doses before age 65 and one dose over age 65 (there should be a minimum of 5 years between vaccinations).

Human Papillomavirus (HPV) Vaccine

Every year, 6.2 million people in the U.S. are infected by Human Papillomavirus (HPV). The route of transmission is sexual contact. Although infected individuals may recover spontaneously, the virus has been associated with cervical cancer and genital warts. Cervical cancer is a devastating malignancy that, in 2004, killed 3850 women

in the U.S. alone. Fortunately, in 2006, the Food and Drug Administration (FDA) granted a license for production of **Human Papillomavirus (HPV) vaccine**. This is an inactivated vaccine that consists of 4 types of HPV: types 16 and 18 (cause 70% of cervical cancer), and types 6 and 11 (cause 90% of genital warts). Since the virus is common in those with significant sexual activity, the best time to get the vaccine is before the first sexual contact. This is important because the vaccine can provide almost 100% protection against HPV infection (types 16, 18, 6, and 11). The vaccine is recommended for females ages 9-26 years. After the initial dose of vaccine, a second dose in 2 months and a third dose in 6 months complete the course of vaccination.

FIGURE 8-9

**Center for Disease Control (CDC) Recommended Vaccine
Schedule for Adults**

Vaccine	Age	Total doses	Note
Hepatitis A	19-65 years and older	2 (second dose at 6-18 months after the first dose)	For certain high-risk groups[1]
Hepatitis B	19-65 years and older	3 (second dose 1-2 and the third dose at 4-6 months after the first dose)	For certain high-risk groups[1]
Human Papillomavirus (HPV)	See Figure 8-8	3	Those ages 23 and below who have not completed the vaccine series may be vaccinated.
Tetanus, Diphtheria, Pertussis (Td/Tdap)	19-65 years and older	1	1 dose Td every 10 years, substitute 1 dose of Tdap for Td
Measles, Mumps, Rubella (MMR)	14-49 years	1-2	Certain high-risk groups[1] should get 1 dose at 50-65 years and older.
Varicella	19-65 years and older	2 doses (the second dose is 4-8 weeks after the first dose)	
Influenza	50-65 years and older	1 dose (annually)	Certain high-risk groups should receive the vaccine between ages 19-49.
Pneumococcal vaccine (polysaccharide)	65 years and older	1	Certain high-risk groups should receive 1-2 doses of the vaccine between ages 50-64 years of age.
Meningococcal	19-65 years and older	1 or more doses	The doses indicated are for certain high-risk groups.[1]
Zoster	60 years and older	1	

(1) On the basis of medical, occupational, life style, or other indications.

Shingles Vaccine

Varicella Zoster Virus (VZV) causes 2 diseases: **chickenpox** in children (common) and adults (rare), and **shingles** (also known as **herpes zoster**) in adults. Individuals who have contracted chickenpox, or were vaccinated against chickenpox, are in danger of developing shingles later in adulthood. What happens is that the dormant virus becomes reactivated due to immunosuppressive diseases (e.g., AIDS), drugs (steroids, chemotherapeutic agents), radiation, stress, and unknown reasons later in life (usually over 50) and causes shingles. The disease manifests with a painful rash and blisters (main symptoms), fever, chills, headaches, and stomach upset. The rash follows a dermatome (the path of a sensory nerve) on one side of the face or the body and may last up to a month. At times, the pain may continue even after resolution of the rash (**post-herpetic neuralgia**). In 2006, the FDA licensed production of the **Varicella-Zoster Vaccine**. This live viral vaccine is recommended for adults 60 years and older who have had chickenpox. The vaccine should not be used in the following conditions:

- A weakened immune system such as in HIV/AIDS, radiation therapy, or chemotherapy (in cancer patients)
- When taking immunosuppressive medication (e.g., steroids)

- Leukemia and lymphoma
- Severe allergy to gelatin, neomycin or any components of the vaccine
- Pregnancy

PASSIVE IMMUNOTHERAPY

Earlier studies in mice and subsequently in humans have shown that immunity can be transferred from one individual to another. Transferring the serum of an immune person with a specific immunity to a pathogen to an unimmune individual can protect against the same pathogen (**Fig. 8-10**).

The passive transfer of such immunity is known as **passive immunotherapy**. The part of the serum that is mainly responsible for the immunity, as discussed earlier, is gamma globulin (the portion of protein, separated by electrophoresis, that contains the majority of antibodies) (**Fig. 8-11**).

A commercial preparation of immunoglobulins, **Immune Globulin Intravenous (IGIV)**, also known as **Intravenous Immunoglobulin (IVIG)**, is the mainstay of therapy for various immunological diseases. IVIG is IgG prepared by sequential steps of fractionation and precipitation of plasma from thousands of donors (up to 10,000). This large donor population has been exposed to various bacteria and contains a myriad of antibodies. The

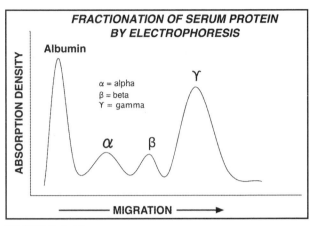

FIGURE 8-11

Food and Drug Administration (FDA) has only a handful of indications for the use of IVIG (**Fig. 8-12**). However, the off-label uses of IVIG cover over 50 conditions.

Among the off-label uses of IVIG, studies report successful treatment of several neurological diseases, including Guillain-Barre syndrome, chronic inflammatory demyelinating polyneuropathy, and multifocal motor neuropathy.

Primary Immunodeficiency and the Use of IVIG

The main indication for IVIG is the management of primary immunodeficiency diseases (PID).

Individuals with primary immunodeficiencies have absent or reduced levels of one or more of the immunoglobulins, or dysfunctional immunoglobulins (unable to react to antigen). Not all primary immunodeficiencies require IVIG. For example, individuals with IgA deficiency may remain asymptomatic or have only occasional mild infections. Therefore, IgA immunodeficiency does not benefit from IVIG. In contrast, individuals with common variable immunodeficiency and X-linked agammaglobulinemia are the best candidates for IVIG therapy. There are several factors to consider in identifying the right candidate for IVIG treatment:

- A history of frequent sinopulmonary infections
- Low levels of serum immunoglobulins
- Low levels of IgG subclasses in spite of normal total IgG
- Low or no change in antibody titer of pneumococcal antibodies post-vaccination.

To test a patient's antibody-producing ability, an individual with low immunoglobulins is vaccinated with

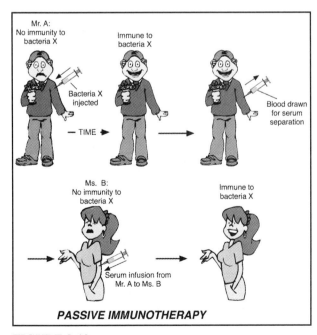

FIGURE 8-10

FIGURE 8-12

FDA Approved Indications for Intravenous Immunoglobulin (IVIG)

Condition	Approved indication
Immunodeficiency	Primary immunodeficiency (PID)
Blood disease	Idiopathic Thrombocytopenic Purpura (ITP)
Transplantation	Bone marrow transplant (graft-versus-host)
Infection	Pediatric HIV
Malignancy	Chronic Lymphocytic Leukemia (CLL)
Vasculitis	Kawasaki syndrome

23-serotype pneumococcal vaccine. The levels of the 23-serotype antibodies are measured before and 4 weeks after vaccination. A normal immunocompetent individual should have a pneumoccocal antibody titer of 2-2$\frac{1}{2}$ times above his/her baseline. Alternatively, *Haemophilus influenza* vaccine may be used to check the function of antibody production before and 4 weeks post-vaccination. The change in titer of antibodies post-vaccination shows how an individual can make antibody to the encapsulated bacteria.

CHAPTER 9.   TRANSPLANTATION

An **implant** is a non-biological object (e.g., saline bag in breast implantation) placed within the body. A **transplant** is a biological object (e.g., hair, skin, heart, finger) transferred from one anatomical site to another. The transplanted material is called a **graft**. The purposes of transplantation vary (**Fig. 9-1**).

TYPES OF GRAFTS

The nomenclature of transplantation is based on the genetic relationship of the donor and recipient (**Fig. 9-2**).

An **autograft** is the transplantation of a graft from one site of the body to another in the same individual (e.g., a skin graft in burn patients). In this type of transplantation, the donor and the recipient are the same person. This type of transplantation has a high success rate because of the lack of immune rejection.

Transplantation between identical twins is known as a **syngeneic graft** (also known as **syngraft** or **isograft**). In this transplant, the genetic makeup of the donor and the recipient is identical.

FIGURE 9-2

Types of Graft

Types of grafts	Description	Example
Autograft	Transplantation from self to self	Skin graft in burn patients
Synergeneic graft (syngraft or isograft)	Transplantation between identical twins	Kidney transplant between identical twin siblings
Allogeneic graft (allograft)	Transplantation between nonidentical individuals of the same species	Blood transfusion between two humans
Xenogeneic	Transplantation between two individuals of different species	Cardiac valves from pig to human

---

FIGURE 9-1

Purposes of Transplantation

Condition	Procedure	Benefit
Advanced cardiomyopathy	Heart transplant	Survival
Thyroidectomy	Transplanting thyroid tissue post-thyroidectomy	Improves thyroid function
Burn (skin)	Skin graft	• Prevents infection • Improves natural look
Renal failure	Kidney transplant	Independence
Mastectomy	Breast implant in breast cancer patient	Cosmetic
Male pattern baldness	Hair transplant	Cosmetic

An **allogeneic** (also known as **allograft**) transplant is one between individuals of the same species who are not identical twins. The donor could be either live or deceased (cadaver). There are some similarities and some differences in genetic makeup of two individuals who are not identical twins. The success rate of this type of graft is significantly lower than autograft and syngeneic transplantation.

A transplant between two individuals of different species (e.g., a human and an animal) is known as a **xenogeneic graft** (also known as **xenograft**).

GRAFT SUCCESS

When a donor and recipient have an identical genetic makeup (i.e., identical twins), the host immune system accepts the graft. When donor and recipient are genetically different (allogeneic graft), the recipient recognizes the incompatibility of the donor and may reject the graft (**graft rejection**). In order to prevent graft rejection, several markers need to be evaluated. One marker is the ABO blood group. As discussed earlier (Chapter 5), the blood group antigens are located on the cell surfaces of red blood cells and other cells, like the vascular endothelium of the graft.

A successful graft requires compatibility between the blood groups of the donor and the recipient. Another marker to evaluate the compatibility of donor and recipient is the HLA similarity between donor and recipient. Several tests, such as the **mixed leukocyte reaction** and **microcytotoxicity test**, are used to identify the right HLA match between donor and recipient.

In addition to matching donor and recipient, the immune system of the recipient should be suppressed (**immunosuppressive medications**) to prevent reaction with the grafts donor's antigen. The problem is that the recipient must take such medications for life and accepts the risk of long-term side effects. Also, the host (the graft recipient) becomes **immunocompromised** (suppressed immunity) and prone to infections, hypertension, and malignancies.

Several immunosuppressive drugs and their role and side effects are summarized in **Fig. 9-3**. They include corticosteroids (anti-inflammatory), cyclosporin A (calcineurin inhibitor; calcineurin is an enzyme that activates NFAT, a transcription factor necessary for expression of several cytokine genes, such as IL-2 and IL-4), tacrolimus (also known as FK 506; calcineurin inhibitor), azathioprine (antiproliferative agent), rapamycin (antibiotic), and interleukin-2 receptor antagonist (monoclonal antibody).

GRAFT REJECTION

Incompatible grafts are eventually rejected, either immediately or slowly. Different categories of rejection include the following (**Fig. 9-4**):

- **Hyperacute rejection.** This type of graft rejection occurs in minutes to hours post-transplantation. The reason for this rejection is the presence of pre-existing host antibodies to the ABO and/or the donor HLA antigens. The host antibodies bind to the vascular endothelium of the graft, activating the complement system, which results in endothelial injury, inflammation, and eventual thrombosis and rejection of the graft. This type of rejection can be prevented by cross-matching the donor and recipient ABO and HLA antigens before transplantation (**Fig. 9-5A**).
- **Acute rejection.** Acute graft rejection takes place days or weeks post-transplantation. Both cell-mediated (CD4+ T cells and CD8+ T cells) and the humoral immune system (B cells) are involved in this form of graft rejection. CD8+ T cells may react to the graft directly and destroy the graft by

---

FIGURE 9-3

Common Immunosuppressive Medications

Medication	Class	Mechanism	Clinical use
Corticosteroids	Anti-inflammatory	Several mechanisms of immunosuppression (e.g., down regulation of proinflammatory cytokines)	• Prevent graft rejection • Treat graft rejection
Cyclosporin A	Calcineurin inhibitor (a fungal metabolite)	Blocks T cell proliferation (Inhibits production of IL-2, an important cytokine in T cell proliferation)	Graft survival
Tacrolimus (also known as FK506)	Antibiotic (macrolide), also calcineurin inhibitor	Same as cyclosporin A	Graft survival
Azathioprine	Antiproliferative agent	Inhibits proliferation of T and B cells	Prevents acute rejection
Rapamycin (also known as sirolimus)	Antibiotic	Inhibits IL-2 signaling that leads to T cell proliferation	Prevents and treats graft rejection
Interleukin-2 receptor antagonist	Monoclonal antibody	Blocks T cell activation (prevents binding of IL-2 to its receptor on T cell surface)	Prevents and treats early graft rejection

---

FIGURE 9-4

Types of Graft Rejection

Types of graft rejection	Rejection time	Type of immune response	Cause of rejection
Hyperacute	Minutes to hours	Humoral immune response	Preexisting antibodies due to repeated blood transfusions (antibodies to MHC antigens on white cells) or repeated pregnancies (antibodies to paternal alloantigens of the fetus)
Acute	Days to weeks	Cell-mediated and humoral immune response	Reaction of T and B cells to the graft antigen, causing destruction of the graft
Chronic	Months to years	Cell-mediated and humoral immune response	Reaction of T and B cells to the graft antigen, causing arteriosclerosis of the graft arterial wall and narrowing and occlusion of the graft blood vessel

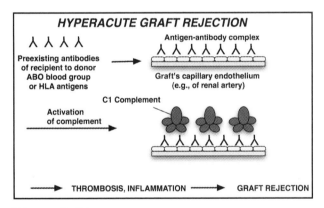

Figure 9-5A

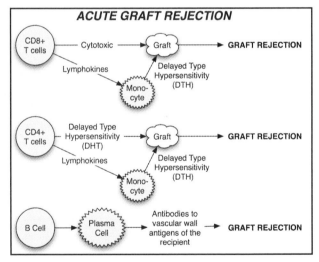

Figure 9-5B

their cytotoxic activity. T cells also release lymphokines, causing stimulation of monocytes. The stimulated monocytes cause delayed type hypersensitivity, which destroys the graft. B cells can also differentiate to plasma cells, producing antibodies to vessel wall antigens, causing rejection of the graft (**Fig. 9-5B**).

- **Chronic rejection.** Chronic rejection occurs months to years post-transplantation. Both cell-mediated and humoral immunity are involved in this graft rejection. Chronic graft rejection manifests as narrowing of the graft vessel wall due to proliferation of intimal smooth muscle, leading to occlusion of the vessel wall (**Fig. 9-5C**).

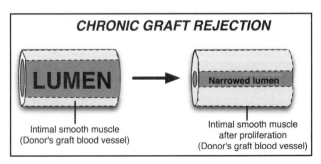

Figure 9-5C

GRAFT-VERSUS-HOST DISEASE

Graft-Versus-Host Disease (**GVHD**) is a type of rejection that is initiated by the **donor** in an immunosuppressed host and is a major complication of bone marrow transplantation. The donor T cells interact with the host's alloantigen (an antigen present in a member of a same species) and starts a cascade of inflammatory reactions, leading to various symptoms and, in severe cases, graft failure. Symptoms may vary based on the target tissues affected. There are two types of GVHD: **acute GVHD** and **chronic GVHD**. Acute GVHD occurs in the first 100 days post-transplantation. The prognosis of acute GVHD depends on the severity of the disease and its response to therapy. Chronic GVHD starts later and lasts for several years. Common symptoms of GVHD include rash, gastrointestinal symptoms (e.g., nausea and diarrhea), and jaundice.

CURRENT PRACTICES IN ORGAN TRANSPLANTATION

Thanks to advanced immunodiagnostic testing, improved surgical procedures, immunosuppressive medications, and organ transplant matching organizations, thousands of organs are successfully transplanted annually. However, thousands more people require organ transplantation yearly and are added to the waiting lists (**Fig. 9-6**).

Some organs are commonly transplanted (e.g., cornea, kidney), but just about every organ and body part can be grafted (**Fig. 9-7**).

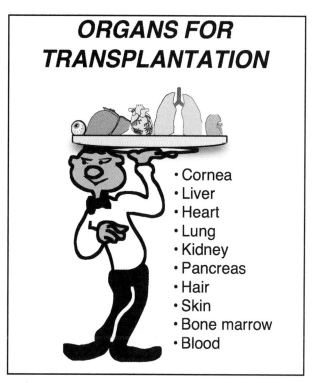

Figure 9-7

The success of transplantation depends on the matching of donor and recipient immunologically (i.e., compatibility of ABO blood group and HLA antigens) and non-immunologically (i.e., gender, age, genetic factors, and others). Organ transplant registry organizations help track availability, the demand for the specific organ, the statistics of successful transplantation, and the match of suitable donors and recipients. Highlights of organ transplantation history in the U.S.A. are summarized in **Fig. 9-8**.

The following are different categories of transplantation based on the organ system:

Hair Transplantation

Type of graft: usually autograft
Type of donor: live donor
Source of graft: usually the occipital area of the same individual (host)
Indications: male pattern baldness
Outcome expectation: restoring natural look
Immunosuppressive medications: not needed
Success: highly successful

Comments. The advancement of hair transplantation has made single, double, or triple hair grafts possible. That is, removing a single, double, or triple hair (with the hair

---

FIGURE 9-6	
The Demand for Organ Transplantation	
Rank	**Organ**
1	Kidney
2	Liver
3	Heart
4	Kidney-pancreas
5	Lung
6	Pancreas
7	Intestine
8	Heart-lung

NOTE: Based on people on waiting lists in the U.S.A. as of August 2008

FIGURE 9-8

Milestones in the History of Organ Transplantation the U.S.A.

Organ	First successful transplant in the U.S.A. (year)	Comment
Kidney	1954	First combined kidney-pancreas transplant was performed in 1966.
Liver	1967	• First split-liver transplant was performed in 1988. • Living donor transplant was performed in 1989.
Pancreas	1968	Less demanding than kidney-pancreas transplant
Heart	1968	First heart transplant globally was performed in South Africa by Dr. Christiaan Barnard in 1967.
Heart and lung (simultaneous)	1981	Not common
Lung transplant (single)	1983	• Double lung transplant performed in 1986 • First successful living donor lung transplant was performed in 1990
Intestine	1987	Not common

---

root) from the donor site (occipital) of the individual and transplanting on the recipient site (the bald area).

Skin Transplantation

Type of graft: autografts, although syngrafts and allografts are possible
Source of graft: any area of the body (usually a non-visible area)
Type of donor: live donor (skin from a skin bank has been used as a biological dressing)
Indications: skin burn
Outcome expectation: coverage of burned area of skin to prevent infection and restore natural look
Immunosuppressive medications: not needed for autograft and syngraft, but needed for allograft
Success: The autograft and syngraft are highly successful; allograft with the use of immunosuppressive medications is also successful.

Blood Transfusion

Blood transfusion is a form of transplantation that preserves life in thousands of recipients every day.
Type of graft: autograft (when blood drawn from an individual is stored for later use, such as surgery), syngraft, allograft
Type of donor: live

Indications: hemorrhage, blood loss anemia
Outcome expectation: restoring life, overcoming anemia
Immunosuppressive medications: not needed
Success: highly successful when matched blood types are used
Comments: The screening of blood for pathogenic microorganisms, such as hepatitis viruses and Human Immunodeficiency Virus (HIV), has made transfusion safe. Individuals should identify their blood type (ABO) and Rh factor for use in blood transfusion in urgent situations.

Heart Transplantation

Dr. Christiaan Barnard performed the first heart transplant in South Africa in 1967. The first successful heart transplant in the U.S.A. was performed in 1968. In 1981, a simultaneous heart-lung transplantation was performed in the U.S.A.
Type of graft: syngraft, allograft, xenograft (in earlier transplantation, a chimpanzee was used as a donor to a human recipient)
Type of donor: brain-dead donor
Indications: idiopathic cardiomyopathy (children and adults), congenital heart disease (children), coronary artery disease (adults)
Outcome expectation: survival, extending healthy life

Immunosuppressive medications: definitely needed
Success: Initial one-year survival was 20% but with inclusion of cyclosporin and more careful screening of donor hearts, the one-year survival rate increased to about 85-90%, and five-year survival rate to about 75-80%.

Lung Transplantation

The first successful single lung transplant and double lung transplant in the U.S.A. were performed in 1983 and 1986 respectively.
Type of graft: syngraft, allograft
Type of donor: brain-dead donor
Indications: cystic fibrosis, emphysema
Outcome expectation: increased quality of life, extended survival
Immunosuppressive medication: needed
Success: generally successful
Comments: It is possible for a donor to donate a lobe of a lung. The lungs may be transplanted in conjunction with a heart.

Liver Transplantation

The first successful liver transplant in the U.S.A. was performed in 1967. The first successful split-liver (partial liver) and the first live donor liver transplant in the U.S.A. were performed in 1988 and 1989 respectively.
Type of graft: syngraft, allograft
Type of donor: cadaver, live donor
Indications: congenital abnormalities, cancer, metabolic disorders, liver failure due to drugs (in children) and cirrhosis (due to a variety of causes, such as alcohol, fatty liver), hepatitis B and C, autoimmune liver diseases, and diseases of the bile ducts (in adults)
Immunosuppressive medications: needed
Success: over 60% first-year survival
Comments: Liver cells can regenerate. Therefore, a liver from a donor can be split and used for two recipients (usually one child and one adult). One of the complications of a liver transplant is graft-versus-host disease (GVHD).

Kidney Transplantation

Kidney transplant is the most common and requested (based on the number of patients on a waiting list) of all organ transplants. After a live donor donates one kidney, the remaining kidney in the donor compensates and takes on the workload of the lost kidney. The first successful kidney and combined kidney-pancreas transplants in the U.S.A. were performed in 1954 and 1966 respectively.
Type of graft: syngraft, allograft

Type of donor: live or cadaver
Clinical use: kidney failure due to a variety of causes, such as diabetes
Immunosuppressive medications: needed
Success: successful
Comments: may be transplanted along with the pancreas

Pancreas Transplantation

The first successful kidney-pancreas transplant in the U.S.A. was performed in 1966. The first single pancreas transplant in the U.S.A. was performed two years later in 1968.
Type of graft: allograft
Type of donor: cadaver
Indications: diabetes mellitus type I
Outcome expectation: production of insulin and prevention of diabetic complications (i.e., nephropathy, neuropathy, and retinopathy)
Immunosuppressive medications: needed
Success: commonly successful
Comments: One of the complications of diabetes mellitus is kidney failure. At times, those in need of a pancreas need a kidney as well and receive a combined kidney-pancreas transplant. Pancreas transplantation may be performed with the whole organ, a segment, or dispersed islets of Langerhans.

Cornea Transplantation

Cornea transplantion is also known as **keratoplasty** or **penetrating keratoplasty** (**PK**). There are approximately 40,000 cornea transplants a year in the U.S.A.
Type of graft: allograft, syngraft
Type of donor: cadaver
Indications: eye injury due to a chemical burn; scarring due to eye infections; thinning and distortion of the cornea, causing **keratoconus**; vision loss due to **Fuchs dystrophy**; corneal edema; corneal ulcer
Outcome expectation: commonly full visual recovery
Immunosuppressive medications: not needed
Success: commonly successful, but there is a 21% rejection
Comments: A newer technique known as **Descemet's Stripping Keratoplasty** (**DESK**) uses a thinner portion of the cornea for transplantation. The advantage is a lesser side effect of astigmatism (nonspherical refraction error).

Bone Marrow Transplantation

Bone marrow transplantation is the second most common transplantation.

Type of graft: autograft, syngeneic, allograft
Type of donor: live donor (the graft is harvested by needle aspiration)
Indications: various diseases, including genetic disease (e.g., Severe Combined Immunodeficiency Disease [SCID], sickle cell anemia, and Wiskott-Aldrich syndrome) as well as malignancies (e.g., acute myelogenous leukemia, acute lymphoblastic leukemia, Hodgkin's and non-Hodgkin's lymphoma).
Outcome expectation: extend life

Immunosuppressive medications: In order to reduce the rate of graft rejection, prior to transplantation, the recipients receive radiation and chemotherapy.
Success: commonly successful
Comments: One of the main problems with bone marrow transplantation is **Graft-Versus-Host Disease (GVHD)**. Administration of immunosuppressive medications to the recipients and treating the donor with specific T cell monoclonal antibody before transplantation may help to prevent GVHD.

CHAPTER 10.   TUMOR IMMUNOLOGY

One function of the human immune system is to recognize and destroy invading tumors. **Tumor immunology** is a branch of immunology that deals with the immune response to tumors.

One can change the morphology and growth properties of animal and human cells **in vitro** (in the laboratory, outside of the body) by using certain chemicals, viruses, and radiation. This results in **transformed cells** with the following characteristics:

- Indefinite growth (immortal)
- Reduced needs for nutrition
- Loss of contact inhibition (able to grow layers over layers)

In the body (**in vivo**), transformed cells proliferate, accumulate, and form a mass known as a **tumor (neoplasm)**. Tumors with limited growth potential and lack of invasiveness into healthy tissues are called **benign tumors**. Tumors that can invade adjacent healthy tissues or travel (via blood or lymphatics) to different sites of the body (**metastasis**) and reside and grow in distant tissues are known as **malignant tumors (cancer)** (Fig. 10-1).

Management of benign tumors consists of surgical removal of the tumor, usually with a good outcome. For malignant tumors, several approaches (such as chemotherapy, radiation, immunotherapy and surgery) have been used with varying success. The stage of the disease (e.g., metastasis) affects treatment outcome (**Fig. 10-2**).

FIGURE 10-2

Features of Benign and Malignant Tumors

Features of a tumor	Benign	Malignant
Growth	Limited	Indefinite (cells are immortal)
Invasiveness into adjacent tissues	-	+
Metastasis	-	+
Treatment	Surgery	Chemotherapy, radiation, immunotherapy, surgery
Prognosis	Good	Uncertain (grave to successful)

CLASSIFICATION OF MALIGNANT TUMORS

A simple way to classify malignant tumors is to divide them into those that originate from hematopoetic stems cells and those that do not. Malignant tumors that do not originate from hematopoetic stem cells are known as **solid organ tumors**. Another way of classifying malignant tumors is based on embryologic **germ cell layer** origin, i.e. ectoderm, mesoderm, or endoderm. **Ectoderm**, the outer layer, gives rise to skin and associated structures. **Endoderm**, the inner layer, gives rise to the gastrointestinal tract and its associated structures. The **mesoderm** lies between ectoderm and endoderm. It gives rise to blood, bone, fat, muscles, and associated structures (**Fig. 10-3**).

For example, the most common malignant tumor, **carcinoma,** derives from either ectoderm or endoderm, while **sarcoma** arises from mesoderm.

Carcinogenesis

How does a normal cell change to a cancer cell? A key step in **carcinogenesis** is genetic alteration of the host DNA. In non-viral-infected cells, a series of spontaneous mutations can transform a normal cell into a cancer cell.

In certain viral-infected hosts, the story is slightly different. The story of viruses and cancers started when U.S.

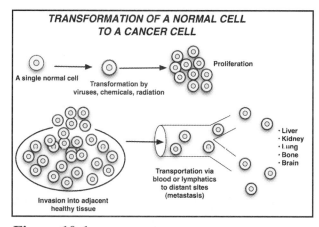

Figure 10-1

GERM CELL LAYERS

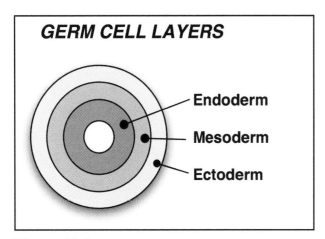

Figure 10-3

pathologist Peyton Rous in the early 1900s removed a connective tissue tumor from a chicken and injected a cell-free extract of it into a healthy chicken; the recipient chicken developed a **sarcoma**. The transforming agent turned out to be a retrovirus (an RNA virus capable of doing reverse transcription) named **Rous Sarcoma Virus (RSV)**. The responsible gene in RSV, capable of transforming a normal cell to a cancer cell, was later designated as *v-Src* (v for virus, src for sarcoma). The importance of this work was recognized half a century later in 1966, when Peyton Rous was awarded a Nobel prize. This gene was the first identified **cancer gene** (also known as **oncogene**, abbreviated *Onc*).

In the 1970s J. Michael Bishop and Harold E. Varmus showed that animals and humans have genes similar to *v-Src*; they called them **proto-oncogenes** (also known as **cellular oncogenes**, abbreviated *C.Onc*). Evidence has confirmed that proto-oncogenes can be converted to oncogenes by one of the following mechanisms:

- **Point mutation.** This is a mutation of a single base in a proto-oncogene. An example is the point mutation of the Ras proto-oncogene.
- **Translocation** occurs when a gene from one location moves to another site of a chromosome and turns on the adjacent gene. An example is translocation of the *c-Myc* oncogene in Burkitt's lymphoma.
- **Amplification** is the production of multiple copies of a gene containing proto-oncogenes, resulting in activation and conversion of proto-oncogenes to oncogenes. An example is the *N-myc* gene in neuroblastoma.

RISK AND PREDISPOSING FACTORS OF MALIGNANCIES

The following factors are known to be risks and predisposing factors of malignancies (**Fig. 10-4**):

- **Genetics** is an important predisposing factor in malignancy. For example, individuals with a family history of colon, breast, and prostate cancer have a higher chance of developing such malignancies than the general population.
- **Geographic areas** may predict the type of specific malignancies. For example, Japan has a relatively high incidence of gastric carcinoma, while Iran has a relatively high incidence of esophageal cancer.

FIGURE 10-4

Risks and Predisposing Factors for Malignancies

Risk factor	Agent or predisposing factor (example)	Malignancy (example)
Genetics	Family history	• Colon cancer • Breast cancer • Prostate cancer
Geography	• Japan • Iran	• Gastric carcinoma • Esophageal cancer
Environment	• Tobacco • Asbestos	• Lung cancer • Mesothelioma
Medications	• Estrogen • Imunosuppressants	• Endometrial cancer • Lymphoma
Viral infections	• Epstein-Barr Virus • Human Immuno-deficiency Virus (HIV)	• Burkitt lymphoma • Kaposi sarcoma
Bacterial infection	*Helicobacter pylori*	Gastric cancer
Ingestants	Tobacco (chewing)	Oropharynx malignancy
Diet	High fat	• Colon cancer • Uterus cancer • Prostate cancer
Radiation	• Ultraviolet light • Ionizing radiation • Isotope radiation	• Skin malignancy • Leukemia • Osteogenic sarcoma

- **Environmental factors.** Tobacco has a strong association with lung cancer. Asbestos (by inhalation) is associated with a specific lung tumor, **mesothelioma**.
- **Medications** such as estrogens may increase the risk of endometrial cancer. Immunosuppressants may make the individual prone to certain types of malignancy (e.g., lymphoma). This is because immunosuppressed individuals cannot recognize and fight against tumor cells as effectively as can immunocompetent individuals.
- Certain **viral infections** have long been associated with malignancies. For example, **Epstein-Barr Virus (EBV)** is associated with **Burkitt lymphoma**, and an increased incidence of **Kaposi sarcoma** is seen in individuals with **Human Immunodeficiency Virus (HIV)**.
- **Bacterial infection** such as *Helicobacter pylori* is associated with gastric cancer.
- **Ingestants.** Tobacco (chewing tobacco) is associated with cancer of the oropharynx.
- **Diet** with a high fat content is a risk factor for certain types of cancer (colon, uterus, and prostate).
- **Radiation** from various sources is associated with malignancies. There are associations between ultraviolet light and skin malignancies; ionizing radiation and leukemia; and isotope radiation and osteogenic sarcoma.

IMMUNE RESPONSE TO TUMORS

In order to prevent **tumorogenesis** (tumor development), the host needs a system to recognize abnormal cell growth and tumors. In addition, the immune system must edit and repair the damaged DNA and destroy the tumor cells.

Tumor recognition. Our immune system can recognize most tumors. In order to recognize tumors, the host searches for an identifier (marker antigens) on tumors. These antigens are either membrane-bound, secretory, or both. Some tumors have specific antigen markers known as **Tumor-Specific Transplantation Antigens (TSTA)** that are specific to tumors and cannot be found in normal cells. Another group of antigen markers are known as **Tumor-Associated Transplantation Antigens (TATA),** which are found during fetal development and in tumor cells (**oncofetal tumor antigens**); they may also be found in lesser amounts in normal adult cells.

The two known oncofetal tumor antigens are **Carcinoembryonic Antigen (CEA)** and **Alpha-Fetoprotein**

(AFP). Carcinoembryonic Antigen (CEA) is a glycoprotein found during fetal development and in various malignancies. It is either a membrane-bound protein, or it can be found in secretory form in peripheral blood. Examples of elevated CEA include colorectal, breast, and lung (squamous) cancer, melanoma, and lymphoma. It is a useful marker to monitor recurrence of colorectal cancer post-treatment. Examples of increased CEA in nonmalignant conditions include chronic cirrhosis, inflammatory bowel disease, pancreatitis, and heavy smoking.

Alpha-Fetoprotein (AFP), an oncofetal antigen, is found during fetal development and in various malignancies. A high level of AFP is found in hepatocellular carcinoma. Elevated levels of AFP are also seen in nonmalignant conditions such as cirrhosis and pregnancy.

There are many other tumor-specific and tumor-associated antigens (**Fig. 10-5**).

Immune Surveillance and Immunoediting

The mechanism that recognizes and eradicates the abnormal cells and tumors is known as **immune surveillance**. This mechanism was proposed in the 1950s, but, without convincing evidence to confirm it, interest waned. Two to

---

FIGURE 10-5

Examples of Tumor Antigen

Tumor marker antigen	Examples of tumors
Carcinoembryonic antigen (CEA)	• Colorectal • Breast • Lung (squamous)
Alpha-Fetoprotein (AFP)	Hepatocellular carcinoma
Beta subunit human chorionic gonadotropin (B-hCG)	Pulmonary (oat and squamous)
MAGE-1, MAGE-3	• Melanoma • Breast • Glioma
Human Papilloma Virus (HPV) E6, E7	Cervical carcinoma
Prostate Specific Antigen (PSA)	Prostate cancer
Tyrosinase	Melanoma

three decades later, however, many studies confirmed the role of immune surveillance in recognizing and eradicating tumors; hence, this theory was revitalized.

We now know that our immune system has a dual role in regard to tumors. One role is to recognize and eradicate tumors (immune surveillance), and the other is to promote tumor formation! Yes, some of the tumors that escape elimination may be selectively chosen to survive and grow. Therefore, a newer theory known as **immunoediting** has been proposed that better describes the role of the immune system and its interaction with tumors. This theory describes three phases, known as the three **E's of immunoediting: Elimination, Equilibrium,** and **Escape**.

Elimination

Elimination (an equivalent step to immune surveillance) is the first phase of immunoediting, in which the host immune system identifies and eradicates tumor. In this phase, both innate and adaptive immunity help to remove the invading tumor. Cytotoxic T cells (CD8+ T cells) have the central role in the elimination phase. Initially, antigen-presenting cells engulf the tumor cells or tumor antigens (**Fig. 10-6**) as follows:

The tumor antigen is broken down, processed, and associated with MHC I molecule, and then displayed on the surface of the antigen-presenting cells (APC). Then the naïve CD8+ cells recognize and bind to the tumor antigen-MHC I molecule; this binding is a signal for activation of the naïve CD8+ cells. The second signal comes from the binding of costimulator (B7) with the CD28 receptor on CD8+ T cell (naïve T cell). The combination of the first and the second activates the naïve CD8+ T cells to become effector cells (cytotoxic CD8+ cells), capable of destroying the tumor cell. Antigen-presenting cells can also present the tumor antigen-associated MHC II molecule to helper T cells (CD4+ T cells). This interaction results in release of several cytokines such as IFN-γ, which activates naïve T cells (CD8+ cells) to become effector cells (CD8+ cytotoxic T cells).

For various reasons, such as reduction or lack of the MHC I expression on tumor cells, cytotoxic T cells may not recognize certain tumor cells. Fortunately, the NK cells can destroy those tumors.

Equilibrium

Equilibrium is the second phase of immunoediting. In spite of all the efforts made in the elimination (immune surveillance) phase, some tumors become resistant to elimination and enter the second phase (**equilibrium**).

Escape

In the **escape** phase, the abnormal and out-of-control growth of tumor cells eventually lead to malignancy.

Killing tumor cells is one way to deal with a neoplasm, but we also have regulating systems to control the growth of normal cells and prevent tumorogenesis. One of these regulating systems is a group of genes known as **tumor suppressor genes** (also known as **anti-oncogenes**, so named because their activation acts the opposite of proto-oncogenes). In addition to regulating normal cell division, these genes repair damaged DNA and also direct the damaged cells to undergo apoptosis (programmed cell death). Any structural changes in these genes (e.g., mutation) leads to abnormal growth of the normal cells, escape, and survival of the damaged DNA.

TUMOR IMMUNOTHERAPY

Tumor immunotherapy, like other types of immunotherapy, is discussed in Chapter 8. It consists of active and passive immunotherapy. In **active immunotherapy**, the reagents used for the therapy stimulate the body's immune system to interact with the tumor. Examples include **tumor vaccines** and cytokines. **Passive tumor immunotherapy** refers to the use of prepared reagents, such as antibodies and cytotoxic T cells, which are introduced into the body to interact with the tumor.

Active Immunotherapy

The vaccines used in active immunotherapy include **preventive** and **therapeutic vaccines (Fig. 10-7)**.

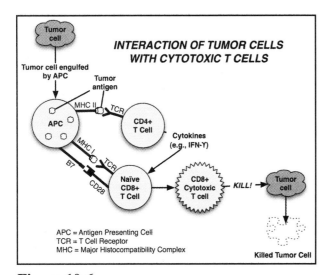

Figure 10-6

FIGURE 10-7

Active Vaccines Approved by the Food and Drug Administration (FDA) for Tumor Immunotherapy

Vaccine	Type of antigen	Vaccine type	Target	Indication
Hepatitis B	Virus	Preventive	Liver	Prevention of liver cancer
Human Papilloma Virus (HPV)	Virus	Preventive	Cervix	Prevention of cervical cancer
Interferon–alpha (IFN-α)	Cytokine	Therapeutic		Therapeutic for:
			Skin	• Melanoma
				• Kaposi sarcoma (AIDS-related)
			Leukocytes	• Chronic myeloid leukemia (CML)
				• Hairy cell leukemia
Interleukin-2 (IL-2)	Cytokine	Therapeutic		Therapeutic for:
			Kidney	• Renal cell carcinoma
			Skin	• Melanoma

Preventive vaccines are used to prevent the host from developing a specific tumor. At this writing, the only Food and Drug Administration (FDA) approved preventive vaccines are hepatitis B vaccine, for preventing hepatocellular carcinoma, and human papilloma virus (HPV) vaccine for preventing cervical cancer.

Generally, vaccines prevent the host from coming down with a specific disease (e.g., MMR vaccine prevents measles, mumps and rubella). **Therapeutic vaccines**, however, differ in that they are used to treat a disease rather than prevent it. The only two cytokines presently approved by the FDA as therapeutic vaccines are **Interferon-alpha (IFN-α)**, and **Interleukin-2 (IL-2)**. More research and data are needed to investigate the potential role of other cytokines such as **Interleukin-12 (IL-12)** and **Granulocyte-Monocyte Colony Stimulating Factor (GM-CSF)** in the treatment of cancer.

- **Interferon-alpha (IFN-α)** is a major cytokine produced by macrophages (also by lymphocytes and dendritic cells). It activates NK cells and increases expression of class I MHC. The FDA has approved IFN-α for treatment of melanoma, hairy cell leukemia, Chronic Myeloid Leukemia (CML), and Kaposi sarcoma (AIDS-related).
- **Interleukin-2 (IL-2)** produced by activated T cells, stimulates the proliferation of lymphocytes (B, T, and NK cells). FDA indications for IL-2 include renal cell carcinoma and melanoma.

Passive Immunotherapy

The best example of **passive immunotherapy** is the use of **monoclonal antibodies**. Since their development in the mid 1970s, monoclonal antibodies have aided diagnosis (e.g., pregnancies, HIV) and improved treatment of many conditions (e.g., psoriasis, arthritis, allergic asthma, cancer, and others). Preparation of monoclonal antibody includes the following steps (**Fig. 10-8**):

- Inject the desired antigen into mice.
- Harvest the mouse spleen B cells containing the specific antibody.
- Fuse the mouse spleen cells with myeloma cells to make them immortal.
- Culture such fused spleen-myeloma cells (known as a **hybridoma**) in a specific culture medium that selects for the growth of the hybridomas only.
- Check the hybridoma with various techniques (e.g., with ELISA) to make sure it produces the desired antibody.
- Prepare a large quantity of the selected hybridoma. Each hybridoma can produce a large quantity of identical antibodies. These antibodies are **monoclonal antibodies**.

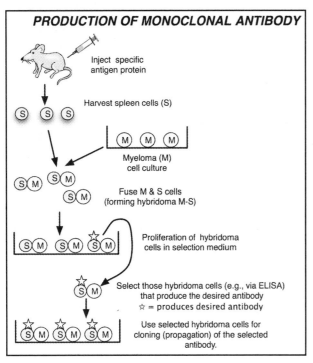

PRODUCTION OF MONOCLONAL ANTIBODY

Inject specific antigen protein

Harvest spleen cells (S)

Myeloma (M) cell culture

Fuse M & S cells (forming hybridoma M-S)

Proliferation of hybridoma cells in selection medium

Select those hybridoma cells (e.g., via ELISA) that produce the desired antibody
☆ = produces desired antibody

Use selected hybridoma cells for cloning (propagation) of the selected antibody.

Figure 10-8

Monoclonal antibodies target specific tumor antigens. Such antibodies can also be conjugated with drugs, toxins, and other therapeutic biological reagents. The uniqueness of monoclonal antibodies is that they are able to go to the target tumor directly and deliver their antitumor action on their own or along with the conjugated drug or toxin. Monoclonal antibodies can cause **apoptosis** (programmed cell death) of the target tumor cells, recruit cells with cytotoxicity (e.g., macrophages) or, after binding to complement, exert direct cytotoxicity. In 1977, the FDA approved the first monoclonal antibody, known as **rituximab**, for treatment of non-Hodgkin's lymphoma. Since then, the FDA has approved several other monoclonal antibodies for treatment of other types of cancer (**Fig. 10-9**).

FIGURE 10-9

A Short List of Monoclonal Antibodies Used in Passive Immunotherapy of Tumors

Type of cancer	Monoclonal antibodies Generic (brand name)	Year of FDA approval
Non-Hodgkin lymphoma	• Rituximab (Rituxan)	1977
	• Ibritumomab tiuxetan (Zevalin)	2002
	• Tositumomab (Bexxar)	2003
Breast	Trastuzumab (Herceptin)	1998
Colorectal	• Bevacizumab (Avastin)	2004
	• Cetuximab (Erbitux)	2004
	• Panitumumab (Vectibix)	2006
Head and neck	Cetuximab (Erbitux)	2006
Acute Myelogenous Leukemia (AML)	Gemtuzumab ozogamicin (Mylotarg)	2000
Chronic Lymphocytic Leukemia (CLL)	Alemtuzumab (Campath)	2001

Index